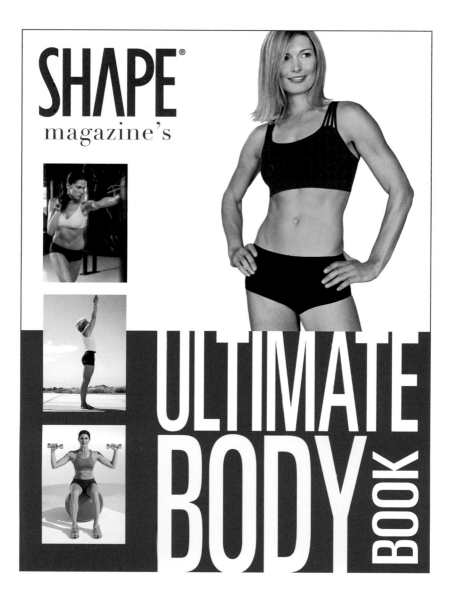

SHAPE®
magazine's

ULTIMATE BODY BOOK

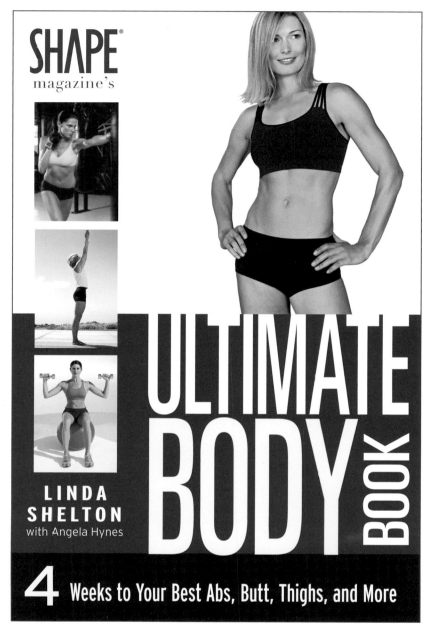

SHAPE®
magazine's

ULTIMATE BODY BOOK

LINDA SHELTON
with Angela Hynes

4 Weeks to Your Best Abs, Butt, Thighs, and More

Produced by The Philip Lief Group, Inc.

HAY HOUSE, INC.
Carlsbad, California
London • Sydney • Johannesburg
Vancouver • Hong Kong

Copyright © 2005 by The Philip Lief Group, Inc., and Weider Publications, Inc.

Published and distributed in the United States by: Hay House, Inc., P.O. Box 5100, Carlsbad, CA 92018-5100 • *Phone:* (760) 431-7695 or (800) 654-5126 • *Fax:* (760) 431-6948 or (800) 650-5115 • www.hayhouse.com • **Published and distributed in Australia by:** Hay House Australia Pty. Ltd., 18/36 Ralph St., Alexandria NSW 2015 • *Phone:* 612-9669-4299 • *Fax:* 612-9669-4144 • www.hayhouse.com.au • **Published and distributed in the United Kingdom by:** Hay House UK, Ltd. • Unit 62, Canalot Studios • 222 Kensal Rd., London W10 5BN • *Phone:* 44-20-8962-1230 • *Fax:* 44-20-8962-1239 • www.hayhouse.co.uk • **Published and distributed in the Republic of South Africa by:** Hay House SA (Pty), Ltd., P.O. Box 990, Witkoppen 2068 • *Phone/Fax:* 27-11-706-6612 • orders@psdprom.co.za • **Distributed in Canada by:** Raincoast • 9050 Shaughnessy St., Vancouver, B.C. V6P 6E5 • *Phone:* (604) 323-7100 • *Fax:* (604) 323-2600

Editorial supervision: Jill Kramer • *Design:* Amy Rose Szalkiewicz

Shape® is a registered trademark of Weider, LLC

Library of Congress Cataloging-in-Publication Data

Shelton, Linda
  Shape magazine's ultimate body book : 4 weeks to your best abs, butt, thighs, and more! / Linda Shelton with Angela Hynes ; produced by the Philip Lief Group, Inc.
    p. cm.
  ISBN-13: 978-1-4019-0708-2 (hardcover)
  ISBN-10: 1-4019-0708-3 (hardcover)
  ISBN-13: 978-1-4019-0709-9 (tradepaper)
  ISBN-10: 1-4019-0709-1 (tradepaper)
  1. Exercise for women. 2. Physical fitness for women. I. Title: Ultimate body book. II. Hynes, Angela. III. Shape magazine. IV. Title.
  GV482.S54 2005
  613.7'1'082--dc22   2005009176

Hardcover **ISBN 13:** 978-1-4019-0708-2 • Hardcover **ISBN 10:** 1-4019-0708-3
Tradepaper **ISBN 13:** 978-1-4019-0709-9 • Tradepaper **ISBN 10:** 1-4019-0709-1

08 07 06 05   4 3 2 1
1st printing, November 2005

Printed in Singapore by Imago

This book is dedicated to the millions of _Shape_
readers in the U.S. and throughout the world.
Your earnest quest for greater well-being has
provided a continued source of inspiration.
May this information contribute to your
wholeness and joy for life.

contents

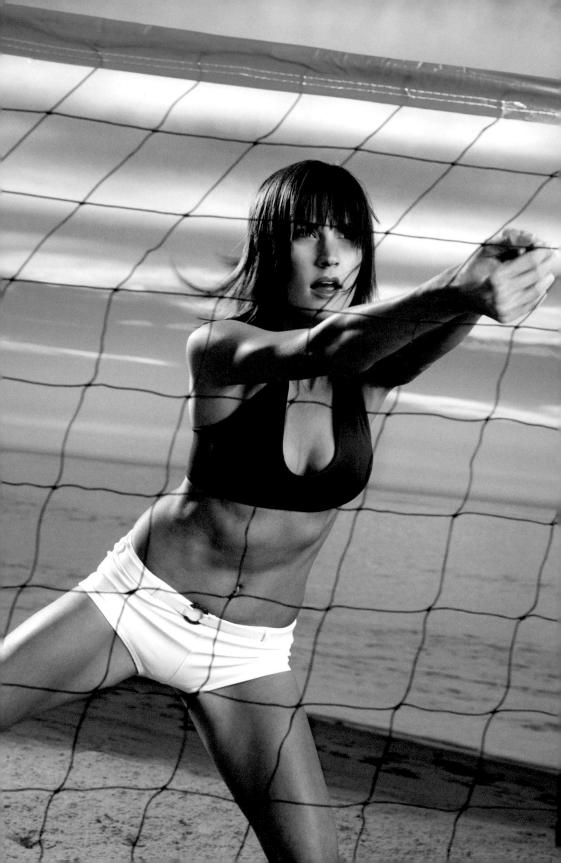

introduction

what defines the ultimate body?

- Do you exercise at least three to five times per week?
- Do you follow an eating plan that contributes to your being lean and full of vitality?
- Are you happy with the way your body looks, given what's healthy and realistic for you?
- Are you happy with how your body performs?
- Do you feel as strong as you'd like to be?
- Do you have the energy you desire?
- Do you feel physically comfortable in your own skin?
- Do you appreciate your body?

If you didn't answer yes to every question (or even if you did), you're in the right place to start making some changes that will get you fit and healthy, and put you on the path toward your Ultimate Body.

But what exactly does that mean? When you hear the words "Ultimate Body," does an image come to mind of a leggy supermodel or a buff athlete? So many of us look at celebrities as role models. But if your ideals are simply *images* of women gleaned from the pages of the glossies, you're setting yourself up for unrealistic and hard-to-sustain goals. The people you see in those pictures are usually young, and often gifted with exceptional physiques and rare metabolisms that allow them to sustain their looks effortlessly. Many photographs have been retouched to make the subjects look flawless, and the super athletes work tirelessly to get those lean and toned bodies. It's often part of their job! They characteristically spend more time than most of us can realistically devote to the pursuit of physical perfection.

When we at *Shape* think "Ultimate Body," we think of *you.* According to the U.S. Department of Health and Human Services, the average American woman is 5'3.7" tall and weighs 152 pounds with a body mass index of 26.3. That's a far cry from the average model, who stands 5'11" and weighs in at 115 pounds. We want you to take a realistic look at your body and accept it—better yet, value and be grateful for it, including its imperfections—and then focus on what's reasonable and possible for you. Set your personal fitness goals accordingly: They might be to lose weight; to target trouble zones like hips, thighs, or abs; or to shake up your workout routine to reach a new level of fitness—in other words, to achieve *your* Ultimate Body.

That's where this book comes in. First, we're going to get you up and moving. According to researchers at the University of California, Berkeley, 86 percent of people don't exercise at all. In a study of nearly 7,000 people, the top three ways in which those 18 and older expend energy are driving (11 percent of daily activity), doing office work (9 percent), and watching television or movies (8.6 percent). In comparison, the top leisure-time physical activities are moderate walking (1 percent), swimming (0.8 percent), and aerobic exercise (0.6 percent).

Is it any wonder that so many of us fall short of being at our peak? Additionally, a sedentary lifestyle breeds self-criticism and a poor body image. But by getting active, you'll start feeling better about your body and yourself, and if you follow our prescription you *will* see visible results in terms of a trimmed-down, toned-up body. Perhaps the best payoff is that you'll feel more energized and positive about your life.

Next we're going to help you eat right to fuel your active lifestyle. And if part of your plan is to lose weight, we'll clue you in on how many calories you need, because there's only one sure formula for permanently dropping fat: exercising more and eating smarter (that is, making better choices to nourish your body and filling yourself up with healthier foods that have fewer total calories).

To get the best results from your exercise and nutrition plans, you need to train smart, and that means applying the right information. In the upcoming chapters, you'll find that in abundance, including: easy-to-follow, illustrated workout plans; data on the physiology of your body; common mistakes or "missteps"; quizzes; frequently asked questions (FAQs) with answers from top fitness professionals; and inspirational stories from women just like you. For example, you'll learn how to do the following:

- Establish your current levels of health and fitness by taking our tests; figure out if you're a beginner, an intermediate, or an advanced exerciser; get tips for your stage of life, whether you're in your 20s or your 40s; and find out if you need to lose weight at all. **(Chapter 1: Your Starting Point)**

- Tone your abs with the ten best techniques so that you'll flatten your midsection and reduce unhealthy belly fat. **(Chapter 2: Awesome Abs)**

- Trim your hips and firm your butt with the top ten exercises, so you'll fit into your jeans better. **(Chapter 3: Toning Your Butt and Hips)**

- Strengthen your legs with the ten most effective moves so that you'll look great in short skirts and have more power to do your cardio weight-loss programs. **(Chapter 4: Training for Tighter Thighs)**

- Sculpt your arms, shoulders, and back with the ten best exercises for helping you feel confident in sleeveless tops, improving your posture, and reducing back pain. **(Chapter 5: A Beautiful Upper Body)**

- Put all of these body-part exercises together in a progressive, specifically designed four-week program for your entire body with variations, depending on whether you're a beginner, an intermediate, or an advanced exerciser. **(Chapter 6: Your Total-Body Program)**

- Increase the intensity of your workouts and beat boredom by using popular tools such as medicine balls and balancing devices. Even the most dedicated exercisers can lose their spark of enthusiasm as well as hit a plateau in terms of their progress. Adding fun tools can help with both problems. **(Chapter 7: Up the Ante with Tools)**

- Explore yoga and Pilates for some serene but surprisingly effective approaches to becoming toned and firm (especially in your core) and flexible all over. Separated by about 5,000 years but kindred in spirit, yoga and Pilates have become 21st-century favorites for achieving strength, balance, and beauty. **(Chapter 8: Yoga and Pilates)**

- Establish great programs filled with cardiovascular exercises—some including moves that will have you playing like a kid—for losing weight and attaining optimal health. We'll also divulge the best-kept secrets for revving up your cardio to burn more calories and making your workouts seem easier. **(Chapter 9: Fat-Burning [and Tush-Toning] Cardio)**

- Stay on track with exercises that you can do at home or on the road with no, or a minimal amount of, equipment. You'll never have to miss your workouts once we eliminate your favorite reason for saying you don't exercise ("no time") by giving you fast, simple routines that make it nonnegotiable. **(Chapter 10: Quick Do-Anywhere [No-Excuses] Workouts)**

- Higher-intensity workouts making use of machines at the gym to help you build more muscle, break through plateaus, and keep you inspired. You've probably heard the axiom "Insanity is doing the same thing over and over and expecting a different outcome"—right? So if you're not regularly introducing more challenging techniques to your workout, how can you expect different body results? Here you'll find those ways to vary your training. **(Chapter 11: Weight-Room Workouts)**

- Workouts with options that you can do in the comfort of your home or at the health club for variety. You can't always get to the gym, and sometimes you just don't want to drag yourself out to battle traffic or bad weather. Now you can keep up with your workout routine at home without missing a beat. Or if you primarily exercise at home, you can hit the gym for a change of scenery and still stick to your program. **(Chapter 12: Programs for Home or Gym)**

- Delicious ways to eat more of what's good for your body, with grocery lists; healthful-cooking techniques; calorie-saving secrets; and loads of delicious recipes for breakfasts, lunches, dinners, desserts, and snacks that you'll look forward to cooking and eating. There are even special recipes to fire you up for your workouts. **(Chapter 13: Eat Smart, Eat Lean)**

Creating the life you want in any area—including achieving your Ultimate Body—requires that you make conscious decisions. You've made a positive one by picking up this book. All you need to do is choose from it what's right for you, and follow through with it every day, step-by-step. As you gain strength and energy, you'll also gain a new appreciation of your body.

Now we're going to let you in on a secret: Women who feel positive about their bodies never seem to obsess about how their bodies *look*. These body-confident individuals have evolved beyond worry about thinner thighs and flatter abs. Instead, they focus on what their bodies can *do*, which opens up a whole new world of possibilities. And that, in the end, is what you'll gain by striving for your Ultimate Body.

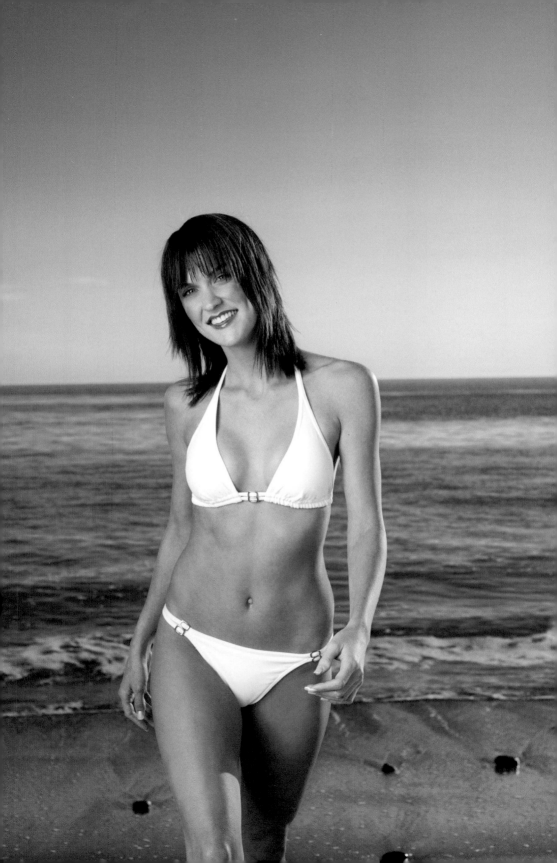

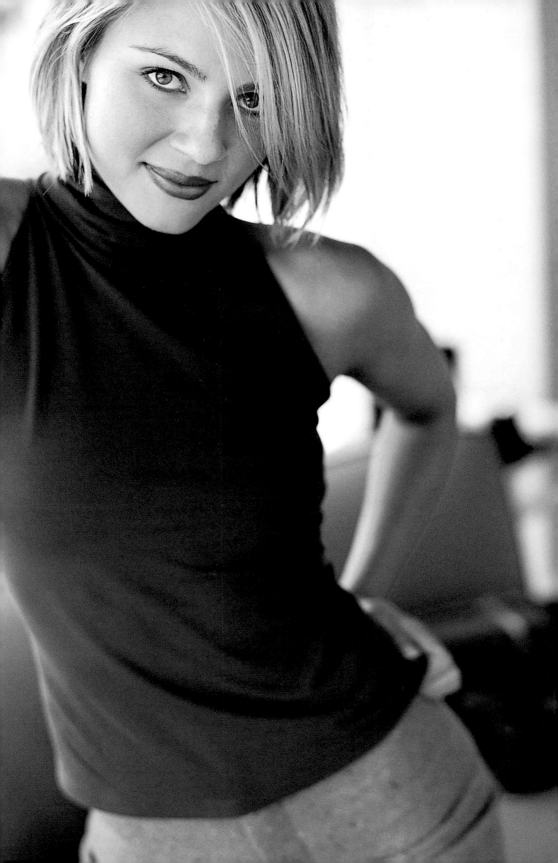

chapter 1

your starting point

Each person picking up this book will be at a different level of health and fitness and will have different goals. What-ever your personal circumstances, you'll find everything you need here to work toward your Ultimate Body—but it will help to know where you're starting from so that you can maximize the information and do the programs that will work best for you. You'll need to be ready both mentally and physically for change.

This Chapter's To-Do List

In this chapter, you'll:

- Make some healthy goals
- Figure out if you're ready for change
- Determine if you're healthy enough to start exercising
- Test your current level of fitness
- Discover if you need to lose weight
- Factor in your age

Your "Real" Ultimate-Body Goal

Many of you will be approaching the programs in this book with a specific goal in mind. You might want to make an entrance at a milestone occasion such as a wedding or reunion, be "bikini-licious" on the beach next summer, or shore up your confidence by looking fabulous when applying for a job or promotion. There's nothing wrong with drawing some motivation from such things, but when you see your body as a fixer-upper that needs a redo before you can appreciate it or enjoy life to its fullest, you're shortchanging yourself. Remember when John Lennon said that "life is what happens to you while you're busy making other plans"? Well, the same idea applies here. Don't miss out on a world of enjoyable activities and relationships by waiting until you've met some self-determined physical ideal (which may not even be realistic).

There's another danger in hitching your plans to a specific event: Even if you hit your target weight or dress size, after that special occasion is over you might fall back into old habits as a "reward." Before you know it, you could be controlled once again by the scale and the mirror, and reproach yourself for relapsing.

Instead of thinking only about one event, shift your focus to the process—try sticking to a regular workout schedule, increasing how much weight you can lift, or seeing how far you can run or cycle. Meeting these action-oriented goals and supporting them with good nutrition, sound sleep, and a healthy lifestyle may manifest a whole new world of appreciation for what you can *do* rather than how you *look*. As you rejoice in small victories such as ten more minutes on the treadmill or another set of reps, you may be surprised to find that you're judging your Ultimate Body in terms of strength, health, energy, and zest for life—and not in numbers on the scale (although a slimmer, firmer body will be a bonus).

Be even more ambitious: Do you want to hike the Appalachian Trail (or part of it), run a 10K or a marathon, or go to Africa and climb Kilimanjaro? Why not choose one such lofty goal? We believe that the purpose of being fit is to do and see more in the world, to feel more alive in your body, and to love your life more. Get going now, seeing and believing that your Ultimate Body is within reach! Start wherever you are, no matter how unfit you believe yourself to be, and take the first step—then the next and the next. Go slow and steady, keeping your sights on the short-term goal right in front of you until your long-term dream gets closer, growing into loving the process all the way.

Putting your intentions and commitment to creating a healthier life in writing—and having a strategy for achieving it—is the first step toward making this a reality. Before you set out on this journey, get a notebook and write down:

- The changes that you want to make in your life
- What the positive outcomes will be upon making them
- What challenges you could encounter
- Your strategy for dealing with those issues
- Who might help you
- Who might try to sabotage you
- How you'll deal with those people who aren't supportive
- Ideas that will help you just in case you get "off course" occasionally
- Rewards you'll give yourself for making progress

But always keep this in mind: There's so much joy to be gained when fitness becomes second nature.

Are You Ready?

The key to making the lasting changes that will lead to your Ultimate Body may surprise you. It's not having grit and determination to take off pounds, get toned, or run a 10K. It's not feeling really, really fed up with being fat and flabby, and it's not even being born with the right genes. It's being truly *ready*.

Take our quiz to test your readiness. Answer "a" or "b" to the following questions based on your current mind-set. (Be honest. Don't choose what you *think* the "correct" answer is.)

1. Most experts agree that losing one to two pounds a week is a healthy goal, and that it takes four to eight weeks to start seeing muscle tone after you begin strength training. How do you feel when you read that?
   a. Encouraged—that sounds doable.
   b. Panicked! I'm going on a vacation in three weeks and need to look great in a bikini.

2. What's your goal?
   a. I want to be at a healthier weight and look toned.
   b. I want to look like I did in college.

3. How would you describe your recent dieting history?
   a. I'm a bit heavier than I'd like to be, but my weight has stayed stable.
   b. I've lost and regained the same amounts over and over.

4. When you look in a full-length mirror, what crosses your mind?
   a. I could stand to lose a few pounds and tone up, but I think I look pretty good.
   b. Full-length mirror—are you kidding?

5. How would your life be different if you achieved your Ultimate Body?
   a. I'd have more confidence to pursue what I want to do.
   b. I'd have a better social life, and my career would improve, too.

6. What's different about your commitment to get in shape this time?
    a. I'm now willing to make some healthy lifestyle changes.
    b. This time I'm really going to stick to my diet.

7. What would you say is primarily responsible for your not being in peak shape?
    a. I overeat and am too sedentary.
    b. I inherited poor genes, so it's tough for me.

8. Do you think that you can work regular exercise into your schedule?
    a. Yes—I have no choice but to make it a priority.
    b. Doubtful—my life is hectic right now, and it's hard to find time.

9. Do you think that you can develop long-term, healthful eating patterns?
    a. Yes—I know it's the only way to safely and permanently lose weight.
    b. I'll do okay until other people tempt me, or the holidays come around.

10. How do you feel about your chances of achieving your Ultimate Body?
    a. I'm confident that I can reach my best body and maintain it.
    b. I secretly doubt that I can stay on the program and reach my ideal fitness level.

If you answered "a" to all of the questions, congratulations! You seem to be ready for lasting change. If you had any "b" answers, you might want to read and apply the following expert tips to help increase the effectiveness of the programs in this book (and even if you answered "a" all around, you'll get some great information here).

1. Get real about your goals. The closer your current weight is to your goal weight, the more realistic your chances of reaching it are, says Timothy G. Lohman, Ph.D., a professor of physiology at the University of Arizona in Tucson. Research shows that most of us see a 10 percent weight loss as doable, while a larger goal can be daunting. Once you've lost 10 percent of your current weight, you can use this achievement as momentum for losing more (if you so desire). Be equally pragmatic about the time frame: A healthy weight loss is one to two pounds each week. Also, make sure to read "Do You Need to Lose Fat?" on page 12.

2. Dump the "magic bullet" approach. Fixating on the idea that there's one perfect way to lose weight or one miracle machine to get you in shape leads to yo-yo dieting. According to David L. Katz, M.D., the director of the Yale-Griffin Prevention Research Center at Yale University School of Medicine, fads are an unfortunate, disheartening diversion. "They seduce you into thinking that if you try them one more time, they really will be magic," he says. As long as you stay distracted, you'll fail to get the message that you need to learn skills and strategies for healthy living.

3. Benefit from your mistakes. Instead of being discouraged by past failures, use them as learning tools. "Think about which specific behaviors helped you in previous weight-loss attempts and which were not particularly helpful," says Anne M. Fletcher, M.S, R.D., who studies people who lose weight and keep it off.

Make two lists: one of activities or actions you stuck with, and another of those you didn't. The first list might include items such as "Get up 15 minutes earlier to eat a good breakfast so I won't be starving by midmorning" or "Arrange to take a walk with a friend at lunchtime." The second list might contain ideas such as "Get up at 5 A.M. every day to go to the gym" or "Never eat dessert."

If you didn't do these last two things before, you probably won't now, and you may get discouraged trying. Concentrate instead on expanding the doable activities. For example, you might get up a bit earlier to pack a healthful lunch or find a more challenging route for your walks.

5. Overcome barriers to exercise. Many women still have difficulty committing to regular exercise. A study at the Saint Louis University School of Public Health in Missouri found that the main reason given is lack of time. "All the women in the study mentioned a scarcity of social support and discomfort with asking for help to make time to exercise," reports Amy Eyler, Ph.D., an assistant professor of community health. They often felt self-imposed guilt about taking time away from family and other responsibilities.

One way to overcome these barriers is to realize that with regular exercise, "you'll be physically and mentally healthier and have more to offer as a companion, mother, employee, and community member, and you'll feel better about yourself," Eyler says.

6. Deal with distractions. It's hard to stay focused on your body when you're worried about your finances, have an intolerable workload, or are struggling in a relationship. Before embarking on any fitness plan, take a hard look at what's likely to interfere with your efforts by sapping your energy and time, then deal with those issues by seeking appropriate professional help (for example, talking to a therapist or financial advisor) and by making lifestyle changes. But don't use this as an excuse not to get started on your Ultimate-Body program.

7. Take responsibility. When you realize that lasting change is in your power and nobody's going to do it for you, you're truly ready for success.

Once you're in the right frame of mind, you need to assess your current state of health and fitness.

Physical Activity Readiness Questionnaire

Physical Activity Readiness
Questionnaire - PAR-Q
(revised 2002)

PAR-Q & YOU

(A Questionnaire for People Aged 15 to 69)

Regular physical activity is fun and healthy, and increasingly more people are starting to become more active every day. Being more active is very safe for most people. However, some people should check with their doctor before they start becoming much more physically active.

If you are planning to become much more physically active than you are now, start by answering the seven questions in the box below. If you are between the ages of 15 and 69, the PAR-Q will tell you if you should check with your doctor before you start. If you are over 69 years of age, and you are not used to being very active, check with your doctor.

Common sense is your best guide when you answer these questions. Please read the questions carefully and answer each one honestly: check YES or NO.

YES	NO		
☐	☐	1.	Has your doctor ever said that you have a heart condition <u>and</u> that you should only do physical activity recommended by a doctor?
☐	☐	2.	Do you feel pain in your chest when you do physical activity?
☐	☐	3.	In the past month, have you had chest pain when you were not doing physical activity?
☐	☐	4.	Do you lose your balance because of dizziness or do you ever lose consciousness?
☐	☐	5.	Do you have a bone or joint problem (for example, back, knee or hip) that could be made worse by a change in your physical activity?
☐	☐	6.	Is your doctor currently prescribing drugs (for example, water pills) for your blood pressure or heart condition?
☐	☐	7.	Do you know of <u>any other reason</u> why you should not do physical activity?

If you answered

YES to one or more questions

Talk with your doctor by phone or in person BEFORE you start becoming much more physically active or BEFORE you have a fitness appraisal. Tell your doctor about the PAR-Q and which questions you answered YES.

- You may be able to do any activity you want — as long as you start slowly and build up gradually. Or, you may need to restrict your activities to those which are safe for you. Talk with your doctor about the kinds of activities you wish to participate in and follow his/her advice.
- Find out which community programs are safe and helpful for you.

NO to all questions

If you answered NO honestly to <u>all</u> PAR-Q questions, you can be reasonably sure that you can:
- start becoming much more physically active – begin slowly and build up gradually. This is the safest and easiest way to go.
- take part in a fitness appraisal – this is an excellent way to determine your basic fitness so that you can plan the best way for you to live actively. It is also highly recommended that you have your blood pressure evaluated. If your reading is over 144/94, talk with your doctor before you start becoming much more physically active.

DELAY BECOMING MUCH MORE ACTIVE:
- if you are not feeling well because of a temporary illness such as a cold or a fever – wait until you feel better; or
- if you are or may be pregnant – talk to your doctor before you start becoming more active.

PLEASE NOTE: If your health changes so that you then answer YES to any of the above questions, tell your fitness or health professional. Ask whether you should change your physical activity plan.

<u>Informed Use of the PAR-Q:</u> The Canadian Society for Exercise Physiology, Health Canada, and their agents assume no liability for persons who undertake physical activity, and if in doubt after completing this questionnaire, consult your doctor prior to physical activity.

No changes permitted. You are encouraged to photocopy the PAR-Q but only if you use the entire form.

NOTE: If the PAR-Q is being given to a person before he or she participates in a physical activity program or a fitness appraisal, this section may be used for legal or administrative purposes.

"I have read, understood and completed this questionnaire. Any questions I had were answered to my full satisfaction."

NAME _____

SIGNATURE _____ DATE_____

SIGNATURE OF PARENT _____ WITNESS _____
or GUARDIAN (for participants under the age of majority)

Note: This physical activity clearance is valid for a maximum of 12 months from the date it is completed and becomes invalid if your condition changes so that you would answer YES to any of the seven questions.

CSEP
SCPE © Canadian Society for Exercise Physiology   Supported by: ◆ Health Santé
                                                              Canada Canada

What's Your Level of Fitness?

If you answered no to the questions in the Physical Activity Readiness Questionnaire (or if you answered yes and have been cleared by your doctor to begin an exercise program), next you'll want to find out how fit you are. This will determine whether you should start with our beginner, intermediate, or advanced programs. You'll discover where your weaknesses lie and which of our workout plans will best help you meet your goals. Retake the tests after a month of working out. If you've followed the programs, you should see a noticeable improvement in your scores, and feel more energized and confident about your abilities as you progress.

Strength

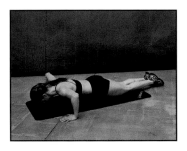

1. Upper-body test: Do as many bent-knee push-ups as you can with good form (no time limit).

Kneel with hands just ahead of shoulders, arms straight, and body forming one straight line from head to hips. Bend elbows to lower body until they're even with shoulders and your chest is about three inches from floor (shown), then straighten arms to push back up to the starting position.

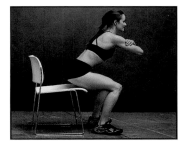

2. Lower-body test: Do as many chair squats as you can with good form (no time limit).

Stand in front of a sturdy chair, feet hip-width apart. Cross arms over chest. Keeping body weight over heels, lower torso (shown) until the backs of your thighs touch the chair seat. Take four seconds to lower and two seconds to stand.

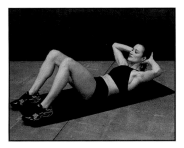

3. Abdominal test: Do as many crunches as you can in one minute, using good form.

Lie faceup with knees bent and feet flat on the floor. Place hands behind head, fingers touching but not clasped. Curl head, neck, and shoulders up until shoulder blades clear the floor (shown), then lower shoulders to floor.

Cardio

The Cooper Institute's Aerobic Fitness Test: Time yourself as you run, jog, or walk for one and a half miles on flat terrain (outdoors or on a treadmill). If you can't run the whole way, start off walking and gradually pick up the pace. Do your best, but don't overexert yourself. Before and after the test, be sure to walk for several minutes to let your body warm up and cool down. Wait at least two hours after eating to take this test.

YOUR RESULTS

Upper Body

[   ] Number of push-ups

How I felt afterward _____

_____

Abdominals

[   ] Number of crunches

How I felt afterward _____

_____

Lower Body

[   ] Number of chair squats

How I felt afterward _____

_____

Cardio

[   ] Time

How I felt afterward _____

_____

Interpreting the Numbers

	Upper-Body Strength (push-ups)	Lower-Body Strength (chair squats)	Abdominal Strength (crunches)	Walk/Run Time (cardio)
Excellent	33 or more	25 or more	48 or more	Below 12:50
Good	22–32	20–24	37–47	12:51–14:23
Average	10–21	15–19	25–36	*
Fair	0–9	10–14	13–24	14:24–15:25
Poor	0	0–9	0–13	Above 15:26

This data provides a range of scores for the average woman. If your scores fall in the Poor category, you're a **beginner**. Those whose numbers are Fair or in the lower ranges of Average are probably **intermediate** exercisers. If you got an Excellent or in the upper range of Good, you're likely an **advanced** exerciser.

You also need to take your age into consideration. Roughly speaking, women ages 20–29 should be aiming at the higher end of each category, women 30–39 at the middle range, and women over 40 at the lower end.

* The Cooper Institute does not use this rating in its aerobic-fitness test.

If You Took a Break from Exercising . . .

You might have picked up this book because you want to get back into shape after taking a break. How you restart an exercise program depends on how long it's been since you last worked out regularly, says Keli Roberts, group fitness manager of Equinox Fitness Club in Pasadena, California. Here's her advice, based on how long you've been away.

- **Two years:** "You're a beginner," says Roberts. You probably have poor aerobic conditioning, muscle tone, and flexibility, so follow our instructions for beginners. Work out at a low to moderate intensity until you feel like your old self again, and expect to experience some muscle soreness.

- **Two months:** You've lost quite a bit of conditioning. You might be tempted to start working out at the level you were at before you stopped, but that would be a mistake and could lead to injury. Roberts recommends taking as long as four weeks to build up to your previous level of activity. Pay particular attention to stretching.

- **Two weeks:** More than likely, you haven't lost any tone and can pick up where you left off. "In fact, if you were training hard before you took the break, you probably will come back stronger," Roberts says. Your body will have had time to rest and recover.

Do You Need to Lose Fat?

One reason you're reading this book might be to lose weight, but don't get fixated on the numbers on your scale: They aren't as important for achieving and maintaining your ideal (that is, healthy) weight as some other numbers are. Without exercise, once you near your 25th birthday, you'll begin to lose lean-muscle mass and replace it with fat at the rate of up to 3 percent per year. By age 60, an inactive woman might weigh the same as she did at age 20 but have twice as much body fat. An excessive amount, especially in areas such as the abdomen, is increasingly recognized as an important risk factor for killers like heart disease and diabetes.

That's why experts now suggest that women ditch weight as a fitness benchmark and look to body composition as a better gauge of how healthy they are.

Assessing Body Fat

Body fat is what's left after you deduct lean tissue (including bones, skin, muscles, and organs) from your overall weight. For optimal fitness, a recent study in *The Physician and Sportsmedicine* points to an ideal body-fat-percentage range between 16 and 25. Less than 12 percent can be dangerous to your health, while more than 32 percent puts you at a high risk for disease and a shorter life span.

Body fat is most precisely assessed by hydrostatic (underwater) weighing, but it may not be readily available, and it can be expensive. The most practical and accurate way to measure is a skin-fold caliper test. This can be up to 96 percent accurate if the average of three times is used, and it's done by an experienced tester. This evaluation is offered at most gyms. However, results for people of color may be skewed by an additional 1 to 3 percent because the formulas most commonly used in health clubs are derived from research performed primarily on white subjects.

If you don't want to go to the trouble and expense of having a body-fat test, you can get a good idea of where you stand by using the calculator on the Shape Up America! Body Fat Lab site at **http://shapeup.org/bodylab**.

You can also buy electronic bathroom scales that measure body fat as well as weight. These can sometimes overestimate, however, so if you're buying one, make sure it has an "athlete mode" for more accuracy. Some health clubs also have devices that measure fat using the same method as these scales—a very weak electrical current (that you can't feel) that detects the amount of fat in your body.

When you're trying to lose body fat, you can also get a rough idea of your progress by tracking your weight and measurements. If your weight is the same but your clothes fit you better and you've lost three inches in your waist, chances are that you're gaining muscle and losing fat.

Waist-to-Hip Ratio

This is a way of determining if your body has too much visceral fat, the risky internal padding around your abdominal organs. Calculate it by dividing your waist measurement by your hip measurement:

1. Measure your waist at its narrowest point (don't squeeze the tape too tight). *Example:* Your waist is 30 inches.

2. Measure your hips at their widest point. *Example:* Your hips measure 40 inches.

3. Divide your waist measurement by your hip measurement. *Example:* 30 ÷ 40 = 0.75. This is your waist-to-hip ratio.

According to the National Institutes of Health, the ideal range is less than 0.8. Between 0.8 and 0.85 is borderline, and above 0.85 is dangerous, since abdominal obesity is linked to heart disease and diabetes. There's some debate as to whether waist measurement alone means more than waist-to-hip ratio, although a recent study at the University of Texas Southwestern confirms that people with large waists and thin thighs have an even higher cardiovascular-disease risk than those who are more obese but store their weight in their lower bodies. To play it safe, experts believe that your waist should be smaller than your hips and less than 35 inches around.

Body Mass Index (BMI)

Calculating BMI, a rough measure that relates body weight to disease risk that's based on height and weight, has become a popular way to determine if you're overweight. You can calculate yours with this simple three-step method:

1. Multiply your weight in pounds by 703.
   Example: You weigh 145 pounds. 145 x 703 = 101,935.

2. Divide the answer by your height in inches.
   Example: If you're 5'4", then 101,935 ÷ 64 = 1,593.

3. Divide the answer again by your height in inches:
   1,593 ÷ 64 = 24.8. This number is your BMI.

The American Institute for Cancer Research encourages a BMI of 18.5 to 25. A BMI above 25, the organization says, puts you at increased risk for cancer, high blood pressure, and heart disease; below 18.5 is usually associated with a lack of lean body mass and may increase your osteoporosis risk.

But your BMI can be misleading. That's because it doesn't take individual circumstances into account—people who are more muscular than normal, or who are thin but unfit. For example, a woman with a "high normal" BMI of 24 or 25 might look healthy but be seriously at risk because she's a sedentary smoker with a family history of heart disease. In her case, body fat is a more accurate barometer of healthy weight.

The Age Factor

If you work out enough, you're much more likely to have a trim, toned, sexy body as long as you also eat healthfully and take care of yourself. But there's more to being active than aesthetic benefits. Regular exercise helps prevent weight gain and bone loss, promotes strong muscles and joints, and has been shown to help stave off some chronic illnesses.

And while it's never too late to get in great shape, you'll be more likely to look and feel your best if you focus on specific exercises at different stages in your life. So whether you're in your 20s, 30s, or 40s, the key to your Ultimate Body (and optimal health) is doing the workout program that's right for you now.

Your 20s

At this point in life, the quest for a sleek and sexy physique typically trumps long-term health concerns. But there are so many reasons to exercise beyond looking good. Both cardio and strength training will keep your body burning calories efficiently, so you won't just be fit and toned, you'll be greatly reducing your risk for obesity-related conditions such as heart disease and diabetes. Those aren't just ailments for old folks: "Type 2 diabetes, once thought of as a disease for middle-aged adults, now affects teenagers and even children," says Palm Beach, Florida–based Reebok University master trainer Joy Prouty. "You can't afford to delay taking care of your body until you're 40." The patterns that you establish now are the key to a lifetime of good habits.

Perform a cardio workout four to six times a week. Push yourself, but be aware of the signs of overtraining, such as fatigue, difficulty sleeping, joint or muscle discomfort, and more than your share of colds. "Doing step aerobics six times a week can do long-term damage," Prouty cautions. Mix up low- and high-impact routines to prevent overuse injuries.

In strength training, focus on core stability—the cornerstone to better posture, control, and performance for every activity you do—as well as your lower body. Develop muscles that are strong and balanced now, and you'll see the payoffs as you age.

Also, use your 20s to explore new sports and exercises in order to find activities you'll love for a lifetime.

Your 30s

The tough reality is that women begin to lose muscle and bone density in their 30s, says kinesiologist James S. Skinner, Ph.D. Some studies have shown that it's possible to achieve slight increases in bone density with exercise, "but it's much harder to increase once you lose it," Skinner notes. "So the issue becomes holding on to what you've got."

Strength is also at issue. Ignore your muscles—particularly the core ones in your torso—and you'll not only find it hard to do everyday tasks and sports, but you'll set yourself up for greater risk of back injury, too.

Don't let lack of time keep you from exercising. Instead, combine strength and cardio training into one circuit workout. Add two to three minutes of marching, walking, running, or rowing between strength moves. Another strategy: Replace one or two long cardio sessions with shorter but more intense workouts each week. Do advanced moves for your abs and back to give you core strength where you need it most and provide an extra challenge as you progress.

Most women in their 30s have frenzied schedules. When your stress peaks, remember that workouts bring emotional balance as well as physical benefits.

Your 40s

"As the years pass, many women settle for weaker muscles, more huffing and puffing, and an expanding waistline," says Prouty. The very time that many fall off the exercise wagon is actually when it's most critical to stay on board. The 40s are when most of us begin to experience the hormonal flux that precedes menopause. This gradual falloff in estrogen means a slowing metabolism, so it's harder to burn calories than it used to be. As if that weren't enough, research shows that fat settles in around a woman's midsection at a faster rate now.

Thankfully, there's a secret weapon: intensity. "Crank up your cardio sessions and you'll get over the metabolic speed bump," says Pamela Peeke, M.D., M.P.H., an assistant professor of medicine at the University of Maryland, Baltimore, and author of *Fight Fat After Forty* and *Body for Life for Women*. And don't forget strength training, which adds bone strength, preserves lean body mass, and boosts muscle so that you can power through your cardio sessions.

Do something active every day, such as a 10- to 15-minute walk, in addition to your three to five days of weekly cardio, and include interval workouts once or twice a week. (Limit jumping and pounding activities if your joints are achy or sore.)

In strength training, target key trouble spots for women in their 40s: the muscles underlying the shoulder blades and those that stabilize the hips and pelvis.

How to Use This Book

Regardless of your level of health and fitness, your current body shape, and your age, there are enough options here for reaching your goals that you're sure to find one or more that you love. But flipping through the pages, you may be confused about which one to choose. And should you follow one plan to completion for four weeks, then switch to a new program—or should you try something new each month? Is it okay to combine plans? The answers depend on your preferences, circumstances, and what you're hoping to achieve.

Whether you should mix it up depends on how fit you are, where you are in your current program, and whether you're seeing results. If you're a beginner, stick with one course from start to finish so that you build a strong base and get into an exercise groove, focusing on your form and increasing your intensity gradually.

But if you're already fit, trying a new plan each month can be a great motivator as well as a boost to your fitness level: Changing helps keep your body from getting too comfortable and staying stuck on a plateau. You also can mix and match, incorporating elements of a new strategy into the one you're already following.

Consider, too, whether you're pleased with the results—are you enjoying the workouts, feeling more fit, and gaining energy? Not every program is for every person. Even though all of ours are fantastic if they're a good fit for you, individuals do respond differently.

You also may not be ready for the course you've chosen; for example, you might not have the necessary balance or control needed to perform the exercises correctly in order to obtain the results promised. If you're not seeing *any* improvement, or you're really feeling uncomfortable with the moves or recommendations, you may consider switching midstream and come back to this plan later on when your body is more ready.

Also, don't dump a program simply because you haven't lost weight as quickly as you'd like. If you have a lot to drop, it won't happen in a month, regardless of which option you choose. This process requires both exercising more and eating less, as well as a healthy dose of patience.

Ultimate Word

In case you need any further encouragement before you start on the programs in this book, here are the top ten reasons why you should get going now:

1. **Your weight:** A program that combines cardio and strength training with sensible eating is the surest way to prevent or reverse weight gain.

2. **Your health:** Regular exercise can help prevent serious health problems, including high blood pressure, type 2 diabetes, heart disease, breast and other cancers, and arthritis.

3. **Your sleep:** Moderate-intensity exercise can improve the quality of your sleep (and more and better sleep can also help you lose weight).

4. **Your bones:** Strength training and some weight-bearing aerobic activities can help prevent osteoporosis and its consequences: thinning, brittle bones; back pain; and stooped posture.

5. **Your brain:** A combination of cardio and strength training not only retards the physical aging of your brain, it also improves your memory and problem-solving abilities.

6. **Your sex life:** Women who exercise regularly reported having sex more often and enjoying it more than their sedentary peers.

7. **Your moods:** Physical activity reduces stress, depression, and anxiety and promotes feelings of well-being.

8. **Your social life:** Joining a gym, working out with a buddy, or training for a race can provide fun and companionship.

9. **Your self-image:** Getting healthy and strong can do wonders for your body image and confidence and that will positively affect all areas of your life.

10. **Your longevity:** Improved muscle strength, flexibility, range of motion, balance, and endurance can help you stay younger longer.

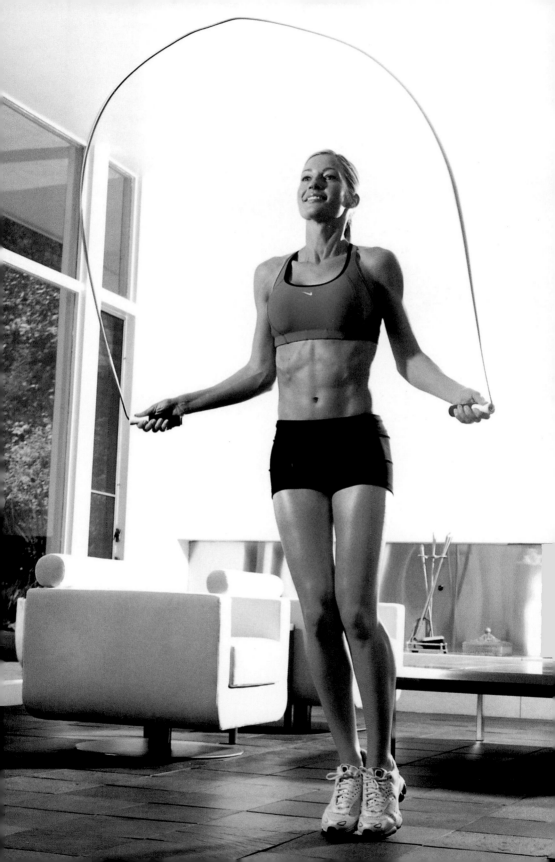

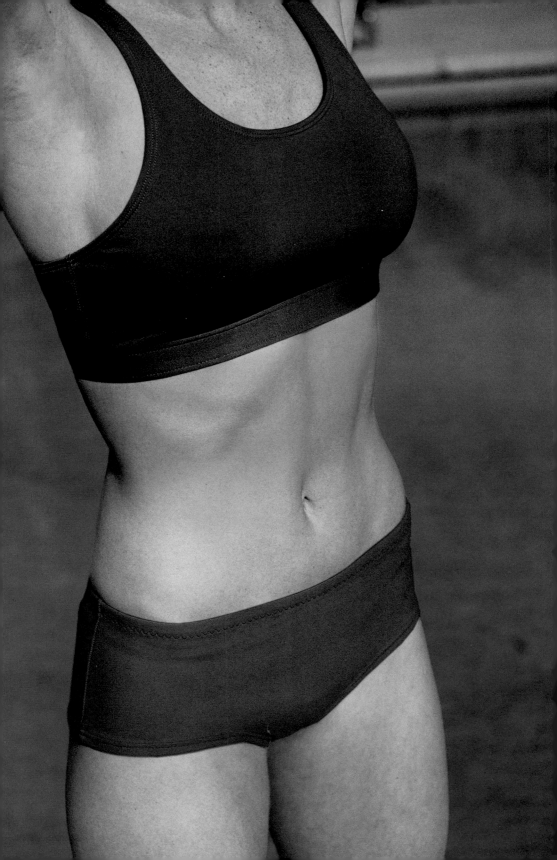

chapter 2

awesome abs

The debate over the best way to flatten your abs is endless. If you were to ask ten trainers what the optimal exercise is for firming your belly, you might get ten different answers. So is there *one* surefire move you can do for the sleek, strong midsection you seek? Unfortunately, the answer is no.

"Stop looking for the one best exercise for abs because it doesn't exist," says Stuart Rugg, Ph.D., chair of the department of kinesiology at Occidental College in Los Angeles. "Abdominal strength and definition come from performing a variety of exercises correctly in a consistent, well-rounded routine."

So with that in mind, what you'll find in this chapter are the most effective moves for awesome abs.

This Chapter's To-Do List

In these pages, you'll learn:

- The myths about training this part of your body
- The ten best moves for strengthening and toning your midriff
- A four-week program that's right for you, whether you're a beginning, intermediate, or advanced exerciser
- What not to do when working your abs

Do You Know the Truth about Ab Training?

You've probably heard most of the hyperbole on ab flattening, from how often you should train to how many reps you have to do. Answer the following questions "true" or "false" to find out if you can separate ab facts from fiction.

1. Strength-training exercises like crunches will get rid of ab fat.

False. Spot reducing isn't possible. While crunches are important for firming and strengthening the abdominals, they won't remove fat. In addition to these exercises, you need to do a total-body strength workout to boost your overall lean-muscle mass, and blast fat and calories with a consistent cardio routine (at least 30 minutes, five days a week, for weight loss). Don't forget to follow a healthy diet, and also realize that genetics plays a part in whether you store more or less fat in your midsection.

2. Sit-ups aren't safe or effective for training your abs.

False. "When done in a controlled manner without the use of momentum, a sit-up is simply a trunk curl taken that much further by the use of the hip flexors, and can be a very effective ab-training exercise," says Wayne Westcott, Ph.D., fitness research director at the South Shore YMCA in Quincy, Massachusetts. So why the bad rap? "People with low-back pain have tight hip flexors and are advised not to do sit-ups because they work the hip flexors a good deal and might exacerbate the issue," Westcott explains. "But really, sit-ups can be done by the majority of the population."

3. If you want to get a firmer, flatter belly, you need to do ab exercises every day.

False. "Although the abs are postural muscles and have a predominance of slow-twitch fibers, which recover quickly from an abundance of work, they are still just like other muscles and need to rest, recover, and rebuild," says certified trainer and fitness author Kurt Brungardt. Train your abs no more than four days a week, on nonconsecutive days.

4. You should train your abs at the end of a workout.

True (and false). There's some validity to the claim that putting your abs last preserves your core strength for the earlier part of your workout: "If you're going to do squats or multimuscle exercises like push-ups or lunges that require a lot of balance, you might want to do abs last so your core is fresh and strong," Brungardt confirms. On the other hand, experts generally agree that you should do ab moves when you're most likely to complete them.

"The danger of always putting abs at the end is that people run out of time and end up never training them," notes Auckland, New Zealand–based certified trainer Kathryn M. Clark.

5. Because the abs are endurance muscles, you have to do hundreds of reps to get results.

False. Abs do have greater endurance than most muscle groups; however, "doing an exercise with proper form, using slow, controlled motions, is an excellent way to maximize results," says Rugg. If you're using correct form, there should be no reason to exceed two or three sets of 25 reps for any ab exercise you do.

"Quality is more important than quantity," Brungardt adds.

The Workouts

There are three levels of workouts that will work all of your ab muscles: beginner, intermediate, and advanced. You'll know which one you should start with by taking our fitness test (if you haven't completed it, go back and do so now). Each program has variations in the moves you'll perform (labeled B, I, and A); the number of sets and reps you'll do; and the amount of weight you'll use (if applicable).

We've given you guidelines to follow for each of the three levels, so read them and make sure that you understand the instructions before you start. Every exercise is numbered, which lets you know where to find the description of how to do it and see it demonstrated in the corresponding photographs. Always warm up with five minutes of light cardio activity; and complete your session by stretching the muscles worked, holding each stretch for 30 seconds without bouncing.

Each workout is a progressive four-week program that you can do either at home or in the gym. In some cases, we've given you options for individual moves that can be done in either place using machines, while some of the other exercises require a dumbbell or weighted ball. If you find a weighted move too difficult, try it first without the weight to perfect your form, and then add the weight when you're ready.

You'll progress from beginner to intermediate to advanced after completing each four-week program, or when you're ready to move on to the next level. Repeat the lower-level programs if your form is poor, you don't feel that you've mastered the moves, or you can't complete the recommended sets or reps with the suggested weight. Even if you're advanced, you might find it beneficial to go back and perform a beginner exercise for variety and to reestablish your form.

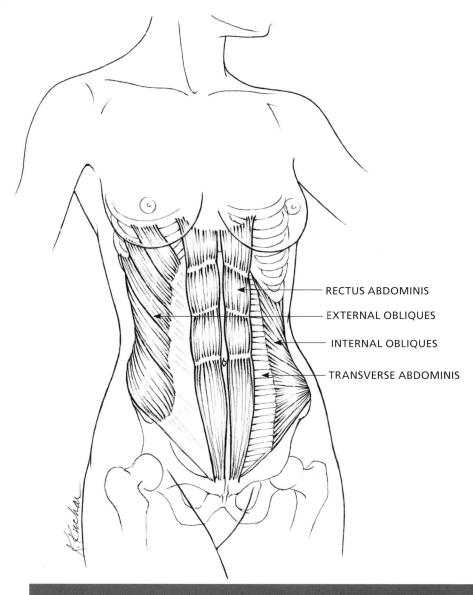

RECTUS ABDOMINIS

EXTERNAL OBLIQUES

INTERNAL OBLIQUES

TRANSVERSE ABDOMINIS

YOUR AB MUSCLES:

The most visible ab muscle, the rectus abdominis, runs from the top of your pubic bone to the sternum (your breastbone). It's attached by connective tissue to the external obliques, which run diagonally from the lower ribs to the middle portion of the upper pelvic bone. The internal obliques run diagonally upward from your pelvis to your lower ribs. The deepest ab muscle, the transverse abdominis, runs horizontally around your middle to attach at your lower back and contracts when the others are used, but can't be worked in isolation.

Beginners

Guidelines: Do these exercises (see page 35 for "The Moves") 2–3 times a week with at least 1 day of rest in between workouts. Perform the suggested number of reps for each move, and rest 45–60 seconds between sets.

Week One

Exercise	Sets	Reps
1. Basic crunch	2	10–12
OR		
2. High cable crunch (gym)	2	10–12
5. Obliques rock and reach	1–2	8–12

Week Two

Exercise	Sets	Reps
4. Stability ball crunch	2	8–12
5. Obliques rock and reach	2	10–15
3. Segmented double crunch	1	8–12

Week Three

Exercise	Sets	Reps
1. Basic crunch	2	12–15
4. Stability ball crunch	2	10–15
OR		
2. High cable crunch (gym)	2	10–15
3. Segmented double crunch	2	8–12

On Days 1 and 3, do one set of each of the exercises in Workout 1 without resting in between. This completes 1 circuit. Day 2, do straight sets for each exercise In Workout 2. Rest if needed, then repeat the circuit 1 or 2 more times.

Exercise	Sets	Reps
Workout 1		
4. Stability ball crunch	1	12–15
1. Basic crunch	1	12–15
5. Obliques rock and reach	1	12–15
Workout 2		
3. Segmented double crunch	2	12–15
OR		
2. High cable crunch (gym)	2	12–15
5. Obliques rock and reach	2	12–15

Intermediate

Guidelines: Do these exercises (see page 35 for "The Moves") 3 times a week with a day of rest in between workouts. You can do these programs as laid out below, resting for 45–60 seconds between each set, or you can do 1 set of each exercise without resting in between. This completes 1 circuit. Rest 45–60 seconds as needed, then repeat the circuit 1 or 2 more times.

Week One

Exercise	Sets	Reps
4. Stability ball crunch	2–3	10–12
6. Weighted bicycle crisscross	2–3	10–12
8. Arabesque bicycle drops	2–3	10–12

Q. What the heck is "neutral posture"?

A. Good posture not only makes you look better, it also prevents injury. Proper alignment—or keeping a "neutral" spine—places the least stress on muscles and joints because you're balancing the tension among all your muscles to maintain your position. To strike a neutral stance, first try out various postural extremes. Here's how:

- Stand with feet hip-width apart.

- Bend knees into a semi-squat, then straight-en legs (but don't lock your knees).

- Tilt pelvis forward and back, making lower back very arched, then very flat. Position pelvis between those extremes so that your tailbone points toward the floor.

- Tighten abs by contracting belly button toward spine without squeezing your butt muscles.

- Lift shoulders toward ears, then lower them, drawing shoulder blades down.

- Round upper back, then squeeze shoulder blades together and lift your chest. Position shoulder blades somewhere between the two extremes.

- Push chin forward and then pull it back until ears are over your shoulders. You're in neutral when ears, shoulders, ribs, hips, knees, and ankles line up.

Exercise	Sets	Reps
3. Segmented double crunch	2–3	12–15
4. Stability ball crunch	2–3	12–15
OR		
2. High cable crunch (gym)	2–3	12–15
5. Obliques rock and reach	2–3	12–15
OR		
7. High-to-low cable chop (gym)	2–3	10–12

Weeks Three and Four

For each workout session, choose from the following programs. You can also do these as circuits, moving from one exercise to the next with no rest, or as straight sets with rest in between each move.

Exercise	Sets	Reps
Workout 1		
9. Forearm plank with knee drops	2–3	10–12
8. Arabesque bicycle drops	2–3	10–12
6. Weighted bicycle crisscross	2–3	12–15
Workout 2		
2. High cable crunch (gym)	2–3	12–15
7. High-to-low cable chop (gym)	2–3	12–15
6. Weighted bicycle crisscross	2–3	12–16
4. Stability ball crunch	2–3	12–15
Workout 3		
3. Segmented double crunch	2–3	12–15
5. Obliques rock and reach	2–3	12–16
8. Arabesque bicycle drops	2–3	16–20
9. Forearm plank with knee drops	2–3	16–20

Advanced

Guidelines: Do these exercises (see page 35 for "The Moves") 3–4 times a week with a day of rest in between workouts. You can do these programs as laid out below, resting for 45–60 seconds between each set, or you can do 1 set of each exercise without resting in between. This completes 1 circuit. Rest 45–60 seconds as needed, then repeat the circuit twice more.

Week One

Exercise	Sets	Reps
4. Stability ball crunch	2–3	12–15
6. Weighted bicycle crisscross	2–3	12–16
8. Arabesque bicycle drops	2–3	12–16
9. Forearm plank with knee drops	2	10–12

Week Two

Exercise	Sets	Reps
3. Segmented double crunch	2–3	12–15
4. Stability ball crunch	2–3	12–15
OR		
2. High cable crunch (gym)	3	12–15
5. Obliques rock and reach	2–3	12–15
OR		
7. High-to-low cable chop (gym)	2–3	10–12
10. Reverse crunch with knee drops	2	8–12

Weeks Three and Four

For each workout session, choose from the following programs. You can also do these as circuits, moving from one exercise to the next with no rest, or as straight sets with rest in between each move.

Exercise	Sets	Reps
Workout 1		
9. Forearm plank with knee drops	2–3	12–16
8. Arabesque bicycle drops	2–3	12–16
6. Weighted bicycle crisscross	2–3	12–16
10. Reverse crunch with knee drops	2–3	12–16
Workout 2		
2. High cable crunch	2–3	12–15
7. High-to-low cable chop (gym)	2–3	12–15
6. Weighted bicycle crisscross	2–3	12–16
10. Reverse crunch with knee drops	2	12–16
4. Stability ball crunch	2–3	12–15
Workout 3		
3. Segmented double crunch	2–3	12–15
5. Obliques rock and reach	2–3	12–15
8. Arabesque bicycle drops	2–3	16–20
9. Forearm plank with knee drops	2–3	16–20
6. Weighted bicycle crisscross	2–3	16–20

Missteps:

- Using momentum instead of your ab muscles to do the work.

- Adding so much weight that you lose your form: When appropriate, use just enough weight to fatigue your muscles.

- Pulling on your neck or dropping your head back when you lift your torso. This takes your neck out of a neutral position and may place strain on it and your shoulders.

- "Hugging" your elbows around your head or clasping your hands, which can place strain on your neck and shoulders.

- Arching your back, pushing your ribs out, or hunching your shoulders as you lift your torso stresses your spine and neck. When lifting your legs, keep your hips stable and back firmly against the floor.

The Moves

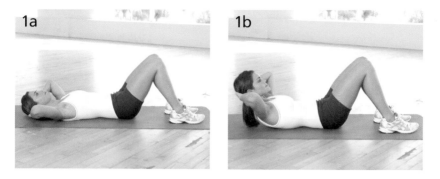

1. Basic crunch (B): Lie faceup on floor, knees bent, and feet flat a comfortable distance from buttocks. Place fingertips unclasped behind head, elbows open. Pull navel in and back toward spine to engage abdominals (a). Inhale, then exhale, lifting head, neck, and shoulder blades upward off the floor in two counts (b). Pause, then lower to start position in 2 counts and repeat.

Strengthens rectus abdominis, external and internal obliques, anc transverse abdominis.

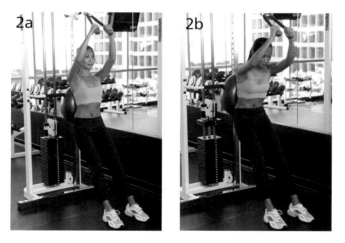

2. High cable crunch (B–I) : Attach a rope to a high-cable pulley then stand against a 45—55 cm stability ball placed between the machine tower and the small of your bac‹, feet hip-width apart, knees slightly bent. Grasp rope with both hands and hold it above your forehead with arms slightly bent, palms facing in. Contract abdominals so that tailbone points toward floor (a). Maintain arm position and flex forward in a crunch motion, bringing ribs to hips without changing hip angle (b). Slowly straighten torso fully to starting position and repeat.

Weight: 20—50 pounds.

Strengthens upper portion of the rectus abdominis, external and internal obliques, and transverse abdominis.

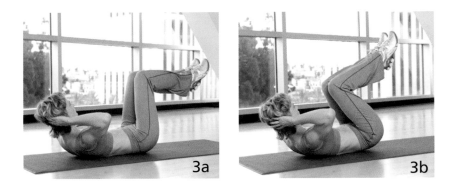

3. Segmented double crunch (B–I): Lie faceup on floor, knees bent in toward chest and aligned with hips, calves parallel to the floor. Place unclasped fingertips behind head, elbows open. Pull navel in toward spine, contracting abs (a). Inhale, then exhale and lift shoulder blades off the floor. Stay lifted and exhale again, lifting hips off floor in a reverse curl (b). Lower hips, keeping legs lifted, then lower torso to the floor and repeat.

Strengthens rectus abdominis, external and internal obliques, and transverse abdominis.

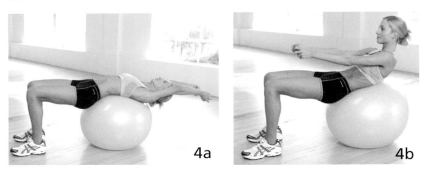

4. Stability ball crunch (B–I): Sit on a stability ball, holding a dumbbell horizontally at your chest with both hands. Walk feet out in front of you, letting ball roll up your spine until your torso is parallel to the floor and supported on the ball from shoulder blades to hips, with head and shoulders off the ball.

Keep feet flat on the floor, knees bent at 90 degrees and aligned over ankles. Contract abs, bringing spine to a neutral position; tuck chin in slightly focusing on a spot just beyond the knees, hips slightly lifted. Extend the dumbbell overhead, arms close to your ears (a). Curl torso upward fluidly, only flexing from the spine, to bring arms up and forward reaching toward your knees (b). Pause, then slowly lower to starting position and repeat.

Weight: 3–8 pounds.

Strengthens rectus abdominis, external and internal obliques, and transverse abdominis.

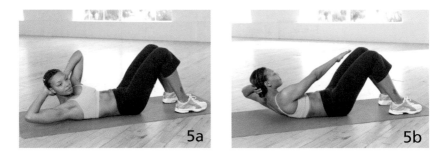

5. Obliques rock and reach (B–I): Lie faceup on floor, knees bent, and feet flat a comfortable distance from buttocks. Place unclasped fingertips behind head, elbows open, and engage abs by pulling your navel in toward spine. Inhale, then exhale, lifting head, neck, and shoulder blades upward off the floor. Holding this lifted position, rotate left elbow toward right knee (a). Stay lifted as you rotate your right shoulder and extend your right arm toward the outside of your left knee (b). Repeat for specified number of reps; lower and rest if needed. Repeat, rotating right elbow to left knee and extending the left arm toward outside of your right knee to complete 1 set.

Strengthens upper fibers of the rectus abdominis, external and internal obliques, and transverse abdominis.

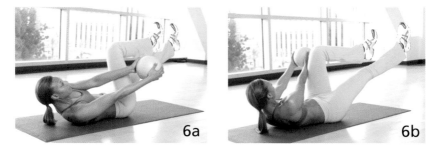

6. Weighted bicycle crisscross (I): Lie faceup with both knees bent and aligned over hips, with calves parallel to floor. Hold a weighted ball in both hands over your chest, elbows bent. Contract abs and lift shoulder blades off floor, but keep lower and middle back firmly on the floor. Chin is level. Straighten left leg toward floor as you extend both arms toward the outside of your right thigh (a). Keep torso lifted and switch your legs, bringing the ball to the outside of your left thigh (b). Repeat, alternating legs and arms to complete the set.

Weight: 2- to 6-pound weighted ball (also known as a "medicine ball").

Strengthens upper fibers of the rectus abdominis, external and internal obliques, and transverse abdominis.

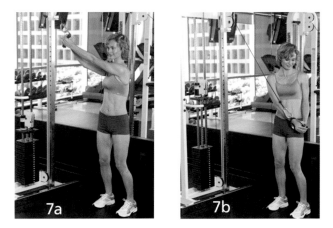

7. High-to-low cable chop (I): Attach a single handle to a high cable pulley, then stand with your right side to the machine. Take 1 large step away from machine and stand with your feet about hip-width apart, knees slightly bent, and toes pointing straight ahead. Hold handle with left hand (underhand) and right hand (overhand) on top of the left, arms extended toward the cable, hips and shoulders square (a). Maintain position and pull handle down and toward the outside of your left hip, letting torso follow the movement, but keeping feet flat and hips square so all movement is in your torso (b). Control the movement as you return to starting position. Do all reps, then switch sides and repeat.

Weight: 10–30 pounds.

Strengthens external and internal obliques, and both rectus and transverse abdominis.

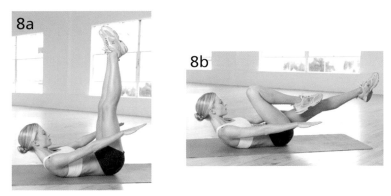

8. Arabesque bicycle drops (I): Lying faceup on floor, extend both legs in the air above your hips, legs and feet together, toes gently pointed, arms at sides. Pull navel in toward spine to engage abs, and lift shoulder blades off floor, extending arms toward legs (a). Maintain lifted position and bend 1 knee in toward chest, lowering other straight leg parallel to floor or as low as you can, while keeping lower back firmly on floor (b). Straighten both legs back up to start position and alternate legs, keeping torso lifted (1 rep per leg).

Strengthens rectus abdominis, and external and internal obliques; uses transverse abdominis as core stabilizer.

Her Ultimate Turning Point

A friend decided to play matchmaker and introduce Timarie Kilsheimer of Maryland to one of her male friends. Before the two met face-to-face, they spent a month talking on the phone and got along well. When they met in person, however, her date took one look at all 250 pounds of Timarie and made an excuse to cut the evening short.

"His rejection shook me up," she says. She determined then and there to lose 100 pounds. By monitoring portions of lean, high-fiber foods; drinking lots of water; and walking regularly, she saw the weight coming off at a rate of 5 pounds a month. When she started strength training 3 or 4 times a week, the loss came even faster. Every time she dropped 10 pounds, she bought a smaller pair of black pants.

"The pants really showed how much weight I was losing," she says. A year and a half later, she surpassed her goal by 10 pounds, losing a total of 110 pounds—and now *she's* the one turning down dates.

Her Best Tip: Take your time doing it so that the weight stays off. The sense of accomplishment will boost your self-esteem.

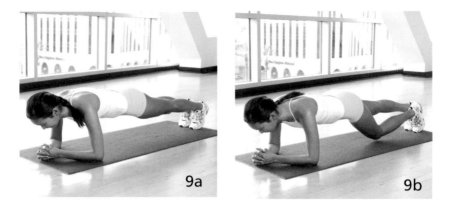

9a · 9b

9. Forearm plank with knee drops (I–A): Kneel with forearms on floor, elbows aligned with shoulders, hands clasped. Extend 1 leg behind you and then the other, so you're supported on the balls of your feet, legs straight and together. Lower hips, pulling abs up and in so that torso forms a straight line from shoulders to heels, hips squared, head and neck aligned with spine (a). Maintain position, and bend 1 knee toward the floor without touching it (b). Straighten leg to starting position and alternate legs, bending and straightening at a fluid, rhythmic pace without letting hips drop or shift side to side. Inhale for 2 knee bends (1 rep), then exhale for 2 knee bends (another rep).

Strengthens rectus abdominis and external and internal obliques; uses transverse abdominis as core stabilizer.

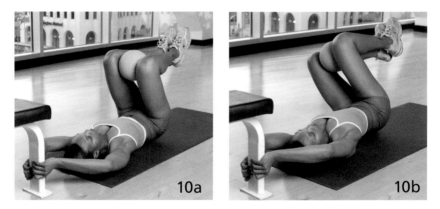

10a · 10b

10. Reverse crunch with knee drops (A): Lie faceup on floor and place a weighted ball between knees, squeezing ball securely. Grasp a stable support behind you, arms straight back behind head, shoulders relaxed and in contact with floor, chest open. Bend knees to align with hips, calves parallel to floor.

Contract abdominals, bringing lower ribs and hips toward each other so that spine is in contact with floor. Inhale, then exhale, using abs to lift hips a few inches off the floor (a). Lower hips to floor, inhale and drop knees toward floor to your left (b). Exhale, bringing legs back to center. Repeat, starting with the lift, then alternate the drops to the right.

Weight: 2- to 6-pound medicine ball.

Strengthens lower fibers of the rectus abdominis, external and internal obliques, and transverse abdominis.

Ultimate Word

While you won't get a tight torso without committing to ab workouts, you can't expect the best results based on exercise alone. Even the most toned muscles won't show if they're hidden under a layer of fat. In addition, belly fat can be particularly bad for your health: Having a waist measurement more than 35 inches for women (37 inches for men) may indicate that you have deep deposits called *visceral fat* that swathe your liver, increasing production of cholesterol and your risk for cardiovascular disease. To keep superficial and deep-belly fat at bay, you need to do the following:

- Blast calories with full-body strength training and cardio (which you'll find in subsequent chapters).

- Learn relaxation techniques such as meditation, deep breathing, and progressive relaxation (consciously tensing and then relaxing your muscles, moving up the body from feet to head) to reduce stress hormones like adrenaline and cortisol that can contribute to deep-belly fat.

- Get 8 hours of sleep, which also helps control stress hormones.

- Eat a diet rich in fish, nuts, whole grains, beans, olive oil, fruits, and veggies, while cutting back on saturated fats and simple carbs such as sugar and white flour.

Now that you've seen the most effective ways to tone your midsection, let's move a bit lower and address some programs designed for your butt and hips.

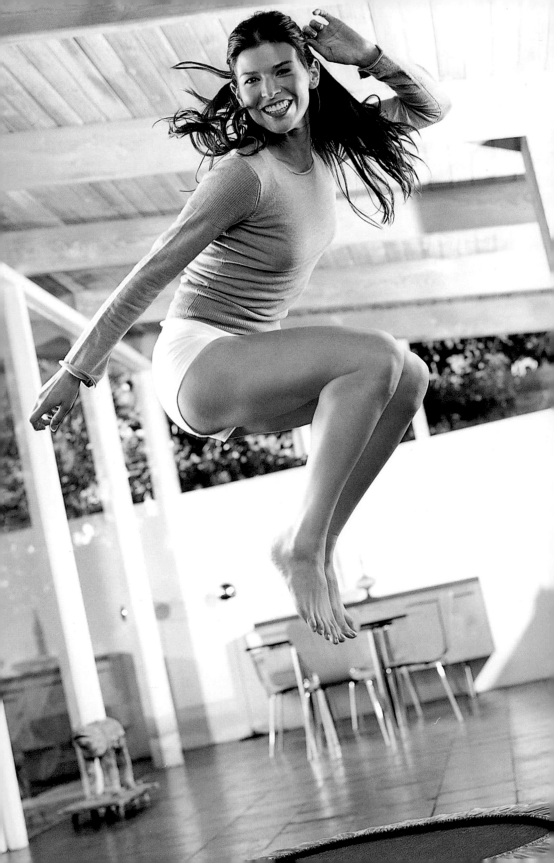

chapter 3

toning your butt and hips

Ask most women what body part they'd most like to perfect, and you'll probably hear a lot about the buttocks—and if not that, it's likely to be the hips. Without a doubt, these are two of our biggest trouble areas, but help is on the way with these supereffective twists on favorite butt and hip exercises that will get your rear in gear and take you one step closer to looking even greater in that pencil skirt or your favorite jeans.

This Chapter's To-Do List

In the following pages, you'll learn:

- The real deal about butt and hip workouts
- The ten best moves for toning and sculpting your rear
- A four-week training program for beginning, intermediate, and advanced exercisers
- What not to do when working your butt and hip muscles

Do You Know the Truth about Butt and Hip Training?

Since so many of you want a backside buff-up, don't you want to know the best way to get it? Answer "true" or "false" to the following questions to see if your knowledge is on the right track.

1. Lunges and squats are all you need to tone your butt.

False. They're both great, effective moves, but "muscles respond much more quickly to a variety of exercises," says Elizabeth Young, physical-therapy aide and instructor at The Cypress Center in Pacific Palisades, California. "If the same exercises are performed over and over again, the dreaded plateau is inevitable." That's why we've given you ten great moves to help you get sleeker hips and a firm derriere.

2. You don't need to do strength training for your butt if you run or cycle.

False. Strength training is far more effective than aerobic exercise for toning your butt, and combining it with cardio is even better. While running is an excellent way to burn calories and strengthen your heart and lungs, says San Diego–based fitness consultant Richard Cotton, M.A., a certification director for the American College of Sports Medicine and chief exercise physiologist of **MyExercisePlan.com,** it won't build muscle mass or strength.

3. If you're already big in the butt, you shouldn't do lower-body workouts because they'll make you even bigger.

False. "There's no reason to avoid any exercise because of your shape," says San Diego–based fitness consultant Ken Baldwin, coordinator of San Diego State University's personal-training certificate program. He confirms that many pear-shaped women fear that moves such as squats and lunges will bulk up their lower bodies. But he explains that these are some of the best exercises you can do to firm and shape this area. Also, because these moves work several large muscle groups at once, they burn more calories than exercises that work by isolation.

When choosing your techniques, don't think about your body shape; instead, focus on whether you're getting a balanced workout. If your major muscle groups don't get equal attention, Baldwin cautions, "Over time you can develop muscle imbalances that can lead to injury." The same goes for your choice of cardio machines. Many women stay away from the stair climber, he says, for the same reason that they avoid squats, but no machine is going to make your butt significantly larger. If you have the type of body that gains muscle easily, you may develop your rear a bit on the stair climber, but in general, cardiovascular exercise does not build much muscle mass.

4. If you don't work out regularly, your glutes will turn into fat, making you *really* broad in the beam.

False. Your muscles may atrophy, but they won't turn into fat. "Muscle and fat are two separate and distinct types of tissue," says Cedric X. Bryant, Ph.D., chief exercise physiologist for the American Council on Exercise. "Muscle can't turn to fat any more than wood can turn into metal. But as muscles shrink because of inactivity, fat can fill the space where the muscles used to be, giving the mistaken impression that the muscles have turned to fat."

With the butt and hip moves contained in this chapter, you'll develop more tone relative to jiggle, and notice more definition. A pound of muscle will take up less area than a pound of fat, so over time you're likely to wear a smaller size of jeans—and look better in them—even though your weight won't necessarily change.

5. Your glutes are such big muscles that you need to work them every day.

False. All muscles need about 48 hours to recover between workouts. If you work the same ones on consecutive days—especially on several consecutive days—you're absolutely overtraining them, no matter what exercises you're performing or which body parts you're working.

"Lifting weights creates microscopic muscle tears, which promote growth and improved strength," says Kara Witzke, Ph.D., an associate professor of exercise science at Norfolk State University in Virginia. "That's a good thing. But if you accumulate microdamage, you end up with large muscle tears. That's not a good thing." If you're working out properly—reaching fatigue after 8 to 12 reps—that part of your body should feel too tired to be challenged on consecutive days. If you find that your muscles feel fresh the day after you worked them, this is a sign that you're not exercising at a high enough intensity to develop significant tone and strength.

The Workouts

Our programs address all of your butt and hip muscles to ensure a balanced workout, so there will be three levels of workouts: beginning, intermediate, and advanced. You'll know which one you should start with by taking our fitness test (if you haven't completed it yet, go back and do so). Each has variations in the moves you'll perform (labeled B, I, and A); the number of sets and reps you'll do; and the amount of weight you'll use (if applicable), or how to make the move more challenging.

We've given you guidelines to follow for each of the three levels, so read them and make sure that you understand the instructions before beginning your workouts. Every exercise is numbered, which lets you know where to find the description of how to do it and see it demonstrated in the corresponding photograph. Always warm up with five minutes of light cardio activity; and complete your workout by stretching the muscles worked, holding each stretch for 30 seconds without bouncing.

Each workout is a progressive four-week program that you can do either at home or in the gym. You'll move from beginner to intermediate to advanced after completing each four-week program, or when you feel that you're ready to go on to the next level. Repeat the lower-level regimens if your form is poor, you

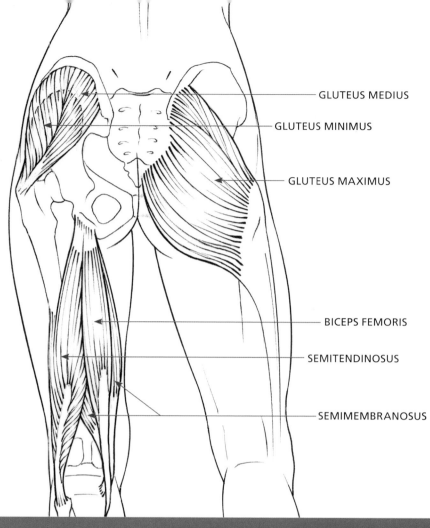

GLUTEUS MEDIUS

GLUTEUS MINIMUS

GLUTEUS MAXIMUS

BICEPS FEMORIS

SEMITENDINOSUS

SEMIMEMBRANOSUS

YOUR BUTT MUSCLES

The gluteus maximus—your largest and outermost buttock muscle—originates on the outer edge of your pelvis and attaches to your rear thighbone. It helps you extend your hips, lift your leg behind you, and turn your thigh outward.

Your primary hip abductor, the gluteus medius, attaches to your pelvis and the top of your thighbone. It helps move your leg out and away from your body with the aid of the gluteus minimus, which is located underneath it, and four other assisting muscles, including the upper fibers of the gluteus maximus. The opposite gluteus medius, along with your adductors (inner-thigh muscles), also works to stabilize your pelvis and keep it from tilting when you're standing on one leg. Finally, the hamstring muscles (biceps femoris, semitendinosus, and semimembranosus), which are on the backs of your thighs, work with the gluteus maximus to extend your hips (move your upper leg to the rear behind you) and are also responsible for bending your knees.

don't feel that you've mastered the moves, or you can't complete the recommended sets or reps with the suggested weight. Even if you're advanced, you might find it beneficial to go back and perform a beginner exercise for variety and to reestablish your form.

Beginners

Guidelines: Do these exercises (see page 55 for "The Moves") 2 to 3 times a week with at least 1 day of rest in between workouts. Perform the suggested number of reps for each move, and rest 45–60 seconds between sets.

Week One

Exercise	Sets	Reps
11. Forearm side-lying lift and extend	2	10–15
12. Reverse froggies	2	8–12

Week Two

Exercise	Sets	Reps
13. Sliding plate rear lunge	1	6–8
11. Forearm side-lying lift and extend	2	10–15

Week Three

Exercise	Sets	Reps
14. One-legged bridge leg extension	1–2	8–12
12. Reverse froggies	2	10–15

Week Four

Exercise	Sets	Reps
13. Sliding plate rear lunge	2	8–12
12. Reverse froggies	2	10–15
14. One-legged bridge leg extension	1–2	8–12

Missteps:

- Letting your knees rotate inward or outward—which will stress both the knee joint and attaching ligaments—rather than aligning them over your feet.

- Stressing your knees by allowing them to move past your toes on lunges or squats.

- Locking your knees when straightening your legs, which can cause knee and back stress.

- Tucking your pelvis under, which prohibits working your butt muscles efficiently.

Intermediate

Guidelines: Do these exercises (see page 55 for "The Moves") 2 to 3 times a week with a day of rest in between workouts. Perform the suggested number of reps for each move, and rest 45–60 seconds between sets. However, where you see the superset, do the 2 exercises grouped together consecutively without pausing between them. Rest 45–60 seconds between supersets.

Week One

Exercise	Sets	Reps
17. Walking lunges	2–3	10–12
18. Step-ups	2–3	10–12
16. Straight legged bar dead lift	2–3	8–12
14. One-legged bridge extension	2–3	10–15

Week Two

Exercise	Sets	Reps
13. Sliding plate rear lunge	2–3	10–12
15. Standing ball rear straight leg lifts	2–3	10–15
12. Reverse froggies	2–3	10–15
16. Straight-legged bar dead lift	2–3	10–15

Week Three

Exercise	Sets	Reps
Superset: *17. Walking lunges*	2–3	8–12
18. Step-ups	2–3	8–12
14. One-legged bridge with leg extension	2–3	10–15

Exercise	Sets	Reps
Superset right leg:		
15. *Standing ball rear straight-leg lifts*	2–3	10–15
13. *Sliding plate rear lunge*	2–3	10–12
Superset left leg:		
15. *Standing ball rear straight-leg lifts*	2–3	10–15
13. *Sliding plate rear lunge*	2–3	10–12

Week Four

Alternate the following workouts.

Exercise	Sets	Reps
Workout 1:		
14. One-legged bridge with leg extension	2	10–15
Superset: 18. *Step-ups*	1	10–15
16. *Straigh-legged bar dead lift*	1	10–15
19. Side lunges with dumbbell reaches	2	10–12
Superset: 18. *Step-ups*	1	10–15
17. *Walking lunges*	1	10–12
Workout 2:		
Superset: 17. *Walking lunges*	2–3	10–12
16. *Straight-legged bar dead lift*	2–3	10–15
Superset right leg:		
19. *Side lunges with dumbbell reach*	2	10–12
15. *Standing ball rear straight-leg lifts*	2	10–12
Superset left leg:		
19. *Side lunges with dumbbell reach*	2	10–12
15. *Standing ball rear straight-leg lifts*	2	10–12
14. One-legged bridge leg extension	2	10–15

Advanced

Guidelines: Do these exercises (see page 55 for "The Moves") 3–4 times a week with a day of rest in between workouts. To superset, do 1 set of each exercise, resting after completing both moves; then repeat them from the beginning. Rest 45–60 seconds between sets and supersets.

Week One

Exercise	Sets	Reps
17. Walking lunges	2–3	12–16
18. Step-ups	2–3	10–15
16. Straight-legged bar dead lift	2–3	10–12
14. One-legged bridge leg extension	2–3	10–15
19. Side lunges with dumbbell reaches	2	10–15

Week Two

Exercise	Sets	Reps
13. Sliding plate rear lunge	2–3	10–16
15. Standing ball rear straight-leg lifts	2–3	12–15
12. Reverse froggies	2–3	12–15
16. Straight-legged bar dead lift	2–3	12–15
20. Curtsy lunge with side-leg lift	2	10–12

Week Three

Exercise	Sets	Reps
Superset: *17. Walking lunges*	2–3	10–12
18. Step-ups	2–3	10–12
14. One-legged bridge leg extension	2–3	12–15

Exercise	Sets	Reps
Superset right leg:		
15. *Standing ball rear straight-leg lifts*	2–3	10–15
13. *Sliding plate rear lunge*	2–3	10–15
Superset left leg:		
15. *Standing ball rear straight-leg lifts*	2–3	10–15
13. *Sliding plate rear lunge*	2–3	10–15
12. Reverse froggies	3	10–12

Week Four

Alternate the following workouts.

Exercise	Sets	Reps
Workout 1		
14. One-legged bridge leg extension	2–3	10–15
Superset: 18. *Step-ups*	2–3	10–15
16. *Straight-legged bar dead lift*	2–3	10–15
16. Side lunges with dumbbell reach	2–3	10–12
Superset: 18. *Step-ups*	2–3	10–15
17. *Walking lunges*	2–3	10–12
19. Standing ball rear straight leg lifts	2–3	10–12
Workout 2		
Superset: 17. *Walking lunges*	2–3	12–15
16. *Straight-legged bar dead lift*	2–3	12–15
Superset right side:		
19. *Side lunges with dumbbell reach*	2–3	10–15
15. *Standing ball rear straight-leg lifts*	2–3	12–15
Superset left side:		
19. *Side lunges with dumbbell reach*	2–3	10–15
15. *Standing ball rear straight-leg lifts*	2–3	12–15
14. One-legged bridge leg extension	2–3	12–15
20. Curtsy lunge with side-leg lift	2–3	10–12

Q. I always hear how important it is to stretch—but is that really true, and if so, why?

A. Stretching helps keep muscles healthy, can make you stronger, and feels great. Specifically:

- Flexibility exercises—when done after a workout or at least after a brief cardio warm-up—help maintain circulation around the joints, keeping muscles healthy where they're most apt to get injured.

- Stretching allows the body to move more efficiently and perform at its peak. According to Jim Wharton, musculoskeletal therapist and owner of Wharton Performance in New York City, muscles begin to shorten as they fatigue during the course of a workout. This impedes your ability to generate speed and power and leads to a less efficient, shorter, more shuffling stride. Stretching keeps muscles elongated, reducing this tendency.

- It can make you stronger. According to research conducted by Wayne Westcott, Ph.D., fitness research director of the South Shore YMCA in Quincy, Massachusetts, stretching after a workout—or even between resistance exercises—can increase strength gains by up to 20 percent.

- It's an incredibly soothing way to connect your mind and body, and it simply feels great!

The Moves

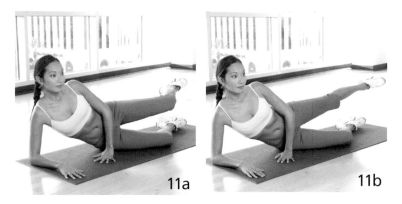

11a 11b

11. Forearm side-lying lift and extend (B): Lie on your right side, propped up on right elbow and forearm, knees slightly bent at a 45-degree angle to your torso. Place left hand on the floor in front of chest for support, hips and shoulders squared, abs pulled in. Keep torso lifted by pressing down through your forearm, and then lift your bent left leg to hip height (a). Straighten left knee directly out to the side without letting leg drop (b). Bend knee then lower to starting position. Repeat for the specified number of reps, then switch legs to complete 1 set.

Weight: 0, or for more of a challenge add 2- to 5-pound ankle weights.

Strengthens upper hips, buttocks, hamstrings, and quadriceps; the abdominals and spine extensors work as stabilizers.

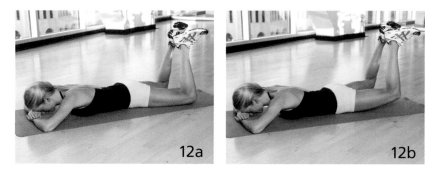

12a 12b

12. Reverse froggies (B–I): Lie facedown on the floor. Place 1 hand over the other and rest forehead on hands, with neck lengthened and chin level. Bend knees and bring heels together, toes and knees turned out, feet flexed with toes pointing toward the floor. Contract abs, drawing tailbone down (a). Keeping heels together and knees open, contract buttocks to lift thighs off ground (b). Pause then release, and lower thighs to the floor. Repeat for the recommended number of reps.

Weight: 0, or for more of a challenge add 2- to 5-pound ankle weights.

Strengthens buttocks and hamstrings.

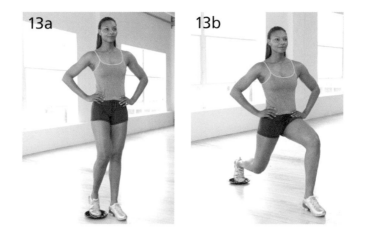

13. Sliding plate rear lunge (B–I): Place the ball of your right foot on a paper plate, then stand with feet about hip-width apart, right knee slightly bent, hands on hips. Pull in abs, bringing spine to a neutral position with chest lifted and shoulders relaxed (a). Keeping abs tight, slide right foot back into a lunge, bending both knees so that left knee aligns with left ankle and right knee approaches the floor with heel lifted (b). Straighten legs, pulling right leg forward and keeping heel lifted. Repeat for specified number of reps before switching sides to complete one set.

Weight: 0, or for more of a challenge hold 8- to 12-pound dumbbells, arms at sides.

Strengthens buttocks, quadriceps, hamstrings, and calves; upper hips and inner thighs, and in both legs work as stabilizers.

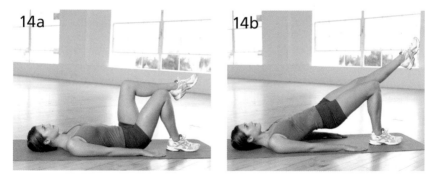

14. One-legged bridge leg extension (B–I): Lie faceup with right knee bent and foot flat on the floor, left knee bent and aligned with hips, calf parallel to the floor, and arms at sides (a). Lift hips up off the floor until torso forms a straight line from shoulders to heel; at the same time straighten left knee, keeping knees at the same height (b). Bend left knee back to starting position and lower hips to the floor. Repeat as recommended, then switch sides to complete 1 set.

Strengthens buttocks, hamstrings, and quadriceps; abdominals, spine extensors, upper hips, and inner thighs work as stabilizers.

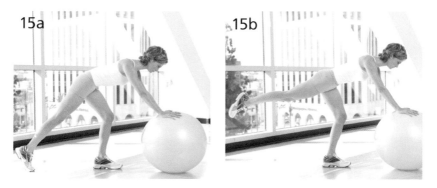

15. Standing ball rear straight-leg lifts (I): Stand in front of a 65-cm stability ball, lean forward from your hips, and place both hands on top of the ball with arms straight. Bend left knee slightly and place toes of right foot behind you on the floor with leg straight. Pull abs in, drawing tailbone down and shoulders blades together (a). Press down on the ball for balance and without leaning sideways or twisting hips, tighten buttocks muscles to lift right leg up to about hip height (B). Pause, then lower toes to the floor. Repeat as recommenced, then switch sides to complete 1 set.

Strengthens buttocks and hamstrings; abdominals and spine extensors work as stabilizers.

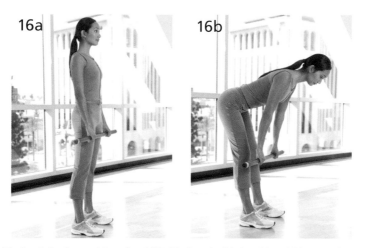

16. Straight-legged bar dead lift (I): Stand with feet hip-width apart, knees straight but not locked. Hold a weighted bar with an overhand grip, slightly wider than shoulder-width, arms hanging straight in front of thighs. Contract abdominals so that spine is in a neutral position (A). Bend forward (like a hinge) at your hips, lowering torso only to the point where you feel your hamstrings tighten; arms will hang down with bar close to body (B). Contract buttocks to straighten back up to an erect position. Repeat for specified number of reps.

Weight: 8- to 25-pound bar.
Strengthens buttocks and hamstrings.

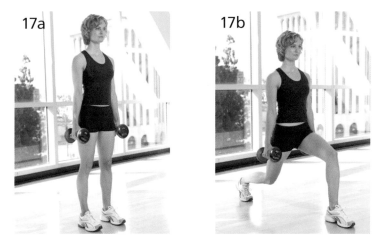

17. Walking lunges (I): Stand with feet hip-width apart and legs straight. Hold a dumbbell in each hand, arms hanging at sides with palms facing in. Pull in abdominals to bring spine to a neutral position with chest lifted and shoulders relaxed (a). Keeping abs tight, take a step forward with left foot, bending both knees so that left knee aligns with left ankle, and right knee approaches the floor with heel lifted (b). Straighten legs as you bring right leg forward and take a step into a lunge. Repeat, alternating legs as you go forward.

Weight: 5–15 pounds in each hand.

Strengthens buttocks, quadriceps, hamstrings, and calves.

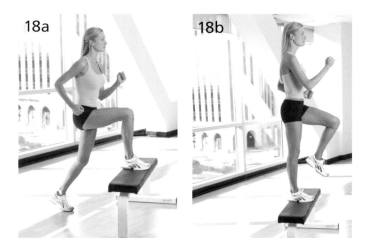

18. Step-ups (I): Stand facing a weight bench or an 8- to 12-inch step with feet hip-width apart, legs straight, but not locked. Contract abdominals to stabilize your spine, drawing shoulder blades together and down. Place right foot on top of bench, bending knee to align with ankle. Keep the ball of left foot on the floor, leg straight and heel lifted, with arms bent in opposition to legs (a). Bend left knee and push off the floor to propel your body upward, straightening right knee so that you're standing on top of bench, lifting left knee to hip height. As you step up, switch your arms (b). Step down onto the floor with left foot, keeping heel lifted, softly bending knee to starting position. Do all reps on one side before switching legs to complete one set.

Strengthens buttocks, quadriceps, hamstrings, calves, upper hips, and inner thighs; abdominals and spine extensors work as stabilizers.

Her Ultimate Turning Point

As a hairdresser on her feet up to ten hours a day and a single mother to a premature baby with health problems, Valerie MacWilliam of British Columbia, Canada, had a demanding schedule. To fuel her long day, she relied on a diet of fast food and caffeinated soda. Three years after her daughter was born, the demands of her stressful life caught up with her: She was 60 pounds overweight and always exhausted. She knew she had to take care of herself if she was to provide the best care for her daughter, so she cut out the soda and began eating healthfully. With no time for gym visits, she used dumbbells and a weight bench to work out at home.

Six months later and 30 pounds lighter, she had a car accident that left her with a torn rotator cuff. Depressed and unable to use her shoulder, she nevertheless kept up with her lower-body strength training and cardio. The accident ended up having a positive dividend: Her work schedule eased up to where she could join a gym. "Regular workouts boosted my spirits, and my depression started to lift," she recalls. Valerie stayed committed to her program until she could resume her upper-body strength-training program, and eventually she shed 30 more pounds.

Her Best Tip: "I usually take Sundays off from my workouts," she says. "It's my day to relax, and it gives my body a chance to recover from my workouts during the week."

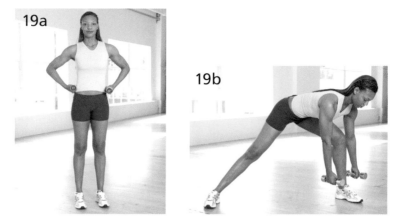

19. Side lunges with dumbbell reaches (I–A): Hold a dumbbell in each hand at your hips and stand with feet slightly apart, legs straight but not locked. Contract abdominals so that spine is neutral, and draw shoulder blades together and down (a). Keeping right leg straight, step sideways with left foot, (about twice hip width), rotating left leg open slightly from the hip so that left toes point out at a 45-degree angle as you bend left knee, aligning it with second toe. As you stabilize your lunging leg, lean forward from hips, keeping spine and neck straight, and lower each dumbbell to either side of left foot (b). Straighten torso to an upright position and push back off of left foot, straightening left leg to starting position. Do all reps on the left or alternate sides, depending on fitness level.

Weight: 5–10 pounds in each hand

Strengthens buttocks, upper hips, quadriceps, hamstrings, and inner thighs of both working and stabilizing legs; abdominals and spine extensors work as stabilizers.

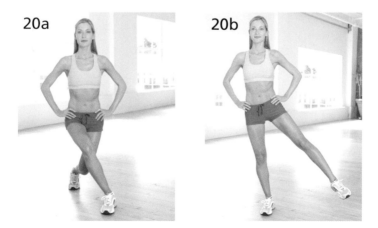

20. Curtsy lunge with side leg lift (A): Stand with feet hip-width apart, legs straight but not locked, and hands on hips. Pull abdominals in, bringing spine to a neutral position with chest lifted and shoulders relaxed. Keep shoulders and hips level and squared to the front as you step backward and on a diagonal with left foot, heel lifted. With torso erect and centered over left thigh, bend both knees, keeping right knee aligned with right ankle and left knee pointing toward the floor (a). Straighten legs and sweep left leg out to the side, maintaining balance (b). Perform reps with left leg, then switch to complete 1 set.

Strengthens buttocks, upper hips, hamstrings, quadriceps, and calves of both working and stabilizing legs; inner thighs, abdominals, and spine extensors work as stabilizers.

Ultimate Word

Many people don't get the full benefits from their butt workouts because their hip-flexor muscles are too tight, says trainer Charleene O'Connor, a private trainer and fitness director at Clay in New York City. You use your hip flexors whenever your walk, run, or perform any action that involves bending your knees or stabilizing your pelvis. Combined with a lot of sitting, this can be a recipe for tight muscles, which can cause you to stick out your butt and arch your lower back, throwing your body out of alignment. When this happens, your buttocks can't contract properly, and other muscles (such as your hamstrings) take over, O'Connor says. Lunge and bridge moves can help open your hip flexors.

Additionally, to ensure proper muscle mechanics and prevent injuries, O'Connor recommends doing this simple stretch after each workout and periodically throughout the day: Standing in a lunge position with your left foot forward, left knee bent and aligned with your left ankle, right leg slightly bent and heel slightly lifted, tilt the lower part of your pelvis forward and contract the right side of your buttocks. Hold for 30 seconds, then switch sides and repeat.

Closely related to your hips and butt are your thighs—and we've devoted the next chapter to helping you get this part of your body into great shape.

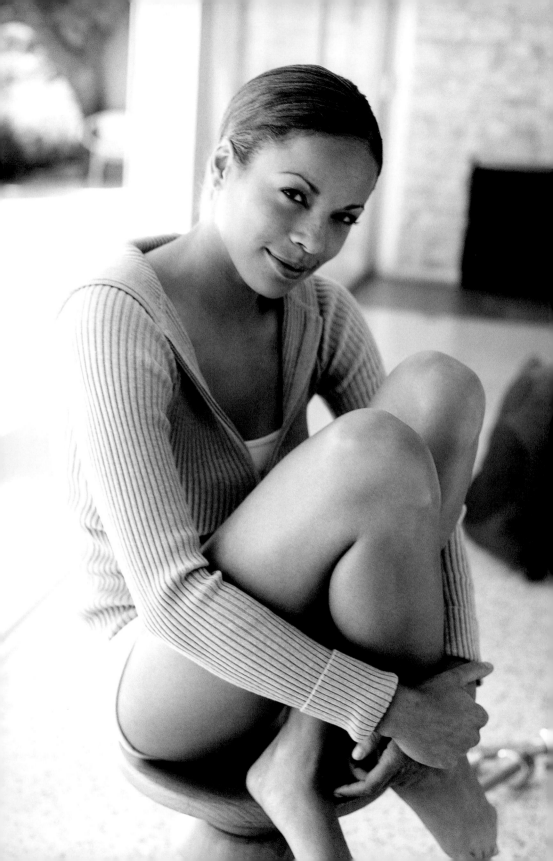

chapter 4

training for tighter thighs

When summer rolls around, do you slip into shorts and thigh-high minis, or do you search for lightweight pants and long skirts that hide your legs—keeping you from fully enjoying summer activities? Well, never fear: After you diligently do the workouts in this chapter, you'll be proud to show off your strong, toned legs! And not only will you be ready for shorts, but you'll also have more power to hike, dance, cycle, and play sports.

This Chapter's To-Do List

In these pages, you'll learn:

- The truth about toning your legs
- The ten best moves for shaping your thighs
- Four-week training programs for beginning, intermediate, and advanced exercisers
- What not to do when working these muscles

Do You Know the Truth about Training Your Thighs?

You might have some misconceptions about this part of your body. Answer "true" or "false" to the following questions to see if you know the road to strong, healthy legs.

1. You can never get rid of saddlebags; they're genetic.

True, to some extent. A pear-shaped body can't be transformed into a string-bean-shaped body, says Los Angeles trainer Ken Alan, a spokesman for the American Council on Exercise, "but you can become a smaller pear." Fat in this area is slow to come off, "so you need to be patient and realistic," he warns.

Lower-body strength training will make your hips more shapely and your leg muscles stronger, giving you more power for your cardio workouts. Activities such as jogging or cycling will significantly boost the number of calories you burn, helping create the calorie deficit necessary for fat loss. (The strength exercises for your chest, back, and shoulders that we present in later chapters will also change your whole body so that it appears more proportional.)

2. Exercise will help reduce the appearance of cellulite on your thighs.

True. Most women develop cellulite to some degree, and how much is often determined by genetics. Here's how it works: Your skin is connected to the underlying muscle by vertical bands of fibrous tissue. Cellulite appears when fat cells bulge up against the top layers of skin, while the fibrous bands pull-down, much like the buttons on a mattress do. "Cellulite is a two-part problem— too little muscle and too much fat," says Wayne Westcott, Ph.D., co-author of *No More Cellulite.* Your first line of attack is to get rid of fat with cardio exercise and healthy eating, but you can also noticeably lessen your skin's dimpling and puckering by toning the underlying muscles for a tighter, smoother appearance. The most effective way to do this is by isolating and fatiguing each muscle. If you needed a good reason to do the moves in this chapter, this may be it.

3. Exercising your thighs will make them bulky instead of slim.

False. Developed muscles actually take up less space than either flabby muscles or the same amount of fat. However, if you're working on your thighs just to trim them down, that's not going to happen either, says Michelle Dozois, co-owner of Breakthru Personal Fitness in Pasadena, California. That doesn't mean that you shouldn't work them. Instead, she says, you need to rethink your approach: Change your focus from thin to strong and functional, and you'll end up with the sleek look you want.

4. You don't need to do additional leg work if you play sports.

False. All serious athletes know that strength training can improve their power and speed. Strong thighs help you with the explosive actions in tennis, kickboxing, volleyball, in-line skating, and skiing. Training this body part can also help prevent injuries, particularly to the knee, since strong quads (along with hamstrings) really help reduce the vulnerability of the knee joint. Soccer players may reduce the risk of ACL (anterior cruciate ligament) injuries, and runners can boost the economy of their movements and help repair the wear and tear on their knees.

5. You shouldn't exercise your thigh muscles if your knees hurt.

False. If you have any pain or injury, you should consult your health-care provider before starting out because you may need to learn some techniques for not putting additional strain on your joints and do some gentle stretching. But according to the Arthritis Foundation, strengthening the muscles around your joints can help stabilize and strengthen them, as well as increasing flexibility and endurance. You may find that strengthening your legs actually decreases knee pain and helps give you the strength and power to make your cardio workouts more effective. The weight loss that can result from doing cardio also helps take stress off of sore knees.

The Workouts

The following pages contain three levels of workouts—beginning, intermediate, and advanced—for toning all of the thigh muscles. You'll know which program you should start with by taking our fitness test (if you haven't completed it yet, go back and do so now). Each has variations in the moves you'll perform (labeled B, I, and A); the number of sets and reps you'll do; and the amount of weight you'll use (if applicable).

We've given you guidelines to follow for each of the three levels, so read them and make sure that you understand the instructions before beginning. Every exercise is numbered, which lets you know where to find the description of how to do it and see it demonstrated in the corresponding photographs. Always warm up with five minutes of light cardio activity, and complete your session by stretching the muscles worked, holding each stretch for 30 seconds without bouncing.

Each workout is a progressive four-week program that you can do either at home or in the gym. You'll move from beginner to intermediate to advanced after completing each four-week program, or when you're ready to go on to the next level. Repeat the lower-level regimens if your form is poor, you don't feel that you've mastered the moves, or you can't complete the recommended sets or reps with the suggested weight. Even if you're advanced, you might find it beneficial to go back and perform a beginner exercise for variety and to reestablish your form.

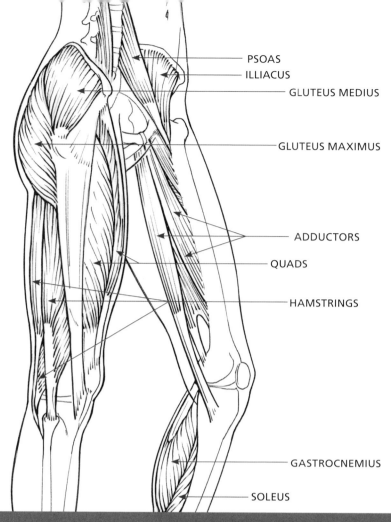

PSOAS
ILLIACUS
GLUTEUS MEDIUS

GLUTEUS MAXIMUS

ADDUCTORS

QUADS

HAMSTRINGS

GASTROCNEMIUS

SOLEUS

YOUR LEG MUSCLES

The inner-thigh muscles include the adductors magnus, brevis, and longus; the gracilis; and the pectineus. The adductors move your legs toward and across the midline of your body, while the gracilis and pectineus are also hip flexors, which bend the hip. The gracilis attaches to the head of the tibia (lower leg bone), and the rest of these muscles attach to your pubis bone and insert on your femur (thighbone). The adductors stabilize and integrate the movements of your legs and pelvis when you walk, run, stand, climb, or lunge.

The hamstring muscles, which are on the rear of your thighs, work with the gluteus maximus to extend your hips (that is, move the upper leg toward the rear) and are also responsible for bending your knees. In contrast, the quadriceps muscles, on the front of your thighs, are involved when you flex your hips to raise your thighs and when you straighten your knees.

There isn't an "outer" thigh muscle, as such. Instead, your hip abductors—a smaller muscle group that's really part of your glutes—form your upper hip and work with your quadriceps to stabilize your knees.

Beginners

Guidelines: Do these exercises (see page 75 for "The Moves") twice a week with at least 1 day of rest in between workouts. To complete a superset, do 1 set of each exercise, resting after both exercises (but not in between them), and then repeat the superset. Perform the suggested number of reps for each move and rest 45–60 seconds between sets and supersets.

Week One

Exercise	Sets	Reps
21. Wall ball squat	2	10–15
24. Lateral shuffle	1–2	8–12

Week Two

Exercise	Sets	Reps
23. Froggies	2	8–12
OR		
22. 3-position leg press (gym)	1	6 each position
24. Lateral shuffle	2	10–15

Week Three

Exercise	Sets	Reps
21. Wall ball squat	2	10–15
23. Froggies	2	10–15
24. Lateral shuffle	2	10–15
OR		
22. 3-position leg press (gym)	2	8–10 each position

Week Four

Exercise	Sets	Reps
24. Lateral shuffle	2	10–15
Superset: *21. Wall ball squat*	2	10–15
23. Froggies	2	10–15

Q. **After you start strength training, how long does it take to gain muscle and see some improvement in tone?**

A. "It takes four to eight weeks of resistance training before you can measure increases in muscles," says exercise physiologist Reed Humphrey, Ph.D., P.T., an associate professor of physical therapy at Idaho State University in Pocatello. But he also notes that how much you'll notice these changes will depend in large part on the amount of fat still covering your muscles.

Another factor is whether you've lifted weights before. "Someone who is deconditioned (i.e., has never strength trained) may see significant changes in as little as four weeks, whereas for someone who's already more fit, it may take six to eight weeks," Humphrey says. Remember that genetics plays a big role in how your body responds to strength training, and keep your expectations realistic. You're not going to look like a model in an exercise equipment infomercial in eight weeks.

For the best results, follow the guidelines in our programs and use weights that are heavy enough to cause fatigue by the end of each set. If you're using weights that are too light, you won't be overloading your muscles sufficiently to see the changes that you're working toward.

Intermediate

Guidelines: This is a progressive 4-week program, either for home or the gym. Do these exercises (see page 75 for "The Moves") 3 times a week with a day of rest in between workouts. To complete a superset, do 1 set of each exercise, resting after both exercises (but not in between them), and then repeat the superset. Rest 45–60 seconds between sets and supersets.

Week One

Exercise	Sets	Reps
25. Plié/relevé	2–3	10–12
28. Skate lunge	2–3	12–15
24. Lateral shuffle	2–3	10–12

Week Two

Exercise	Sets	Reps
27. Front-to-back lunge	2–3	8–12
26. Plié jump and drag	2–3	8–12
OR		
22. 3-position leg press (gym)	2–3	10 each position
23. Froggies	2–3	10–15

Weeks Three and Four

Do **Workout 1** on Days 1 and 3; do **Workout 2** on Day 2.

Exercise	Sets	Reps
Workout 1		
25. Plié/relevé	2–3	12–15
OR		
22. 3-position leg press (gym)	2–3	10 each position

Exercise		Sets	Reps
Superset:	28. *Skate lunge*	2–3	12–15
	24. *Lateral shuffle*	2–3	10–12
23. Froggies		2–3	10–15
Workout 2			
Superset:	27. *Front-to-back lunge*	2–3	10–12
	23. *Froggies*	2–3	10–15
26. Plié jump and drag		2–3	10–12
OR			
29. Balanced low cable squat (gym)		2–3	10–15

Her Turning Point

Deanna Rupp of California was with her three-year-old son at the park when he asked her to go down the playground slide with him. "I climbed to the top and was out of breath when I realized I was too big to fit through the opening to slide down," she recalls. "I was devastated."

With the help of Weight Watchers and a walking program, Deanna lost 30 pounds in three months and then hit a plateau. She talked to her brother-in-law, who'd gotten lean by adding weight training to his routine, and realized that this was exactly what she needed to get going again.

She bought a gym membership and hired a trainer who taught her to use the machines. With this new plan, Deanna's weight loss restarted. She dropped about five pounds a month; and after six months, she reached her target weight of 140 pounds. Now she's a personal trainer helping others reach their goals!

Her Best Tip: Challenge yourself to reach a mini-goal each day, such as doing ten more minutes of cardio or trying a new strength-training exercise.

Advanced

Guidelines: This is a progressive 4-week program, either for home or the gym. Do these exercises (see page 75 for "The Moves") 3 times a week with a day of rest in between workouts. To complete a superset, do 1 set of each exercise, resting after both exercises (but not in between them), and then repeat the superset. Rest 45–60 seconds between sets and supersets.

Week One

Exercise	Sets	Reps
25. Plié/relevé	2–3	12–15
28. Skate lunge	2–3	12–15
24. Lateral shuffle	2–3	10–12
30. Kneeling side planks with leg sweeps	2	6–8

Week Two

Exercise	Sets	Reps
27. Front-to-back lunge	2–3	10–12
29. Balanced low cable squat (gym)	2–3	12–15
26. Plié jump and drag OR	2–3	10–12
22. 3-position leg press (gym)	2–3	10 each position
23. Froggies	2–3	10–15

Weeks Three and Four

Do **Workout 1** on Days 1 and 3; do **Workout 2** on Day 2.

Exercise	Sets	Reps
Workout 1		
25. Plié/relevé	2–3	12–15
OR		
22. 3-position leg press (gym)	2–3	10 each position
Superset: *28. Skate lunge*	2–3	12–15
24. Lateral shuffle	2–3	12–15
Superset: *23. Froggies*	2–3	10–15
30. Kneeling side planks with leg sweeps	2–3	8–12
Workout 2		
Superset *27. Front-to-back lunge*	2–3	10–12
23. Froggies	2–3	10–15
Superset: *26. Plié jump and drag*	2–3	10–12
29. Balanced low cable squat (gym)	2–3	10–12
30. Kneeling side planks with leg sweeps	2–3	8–12

Missteps:

- Flexing your torso forward or leaning backward, which throws off your balance. Doing so makes it difficult to maximize lower-body efficiency.

- Letting your knee "wander" outside or inside of your ankle and toes (or past your toes), as this can change the muscles you're using and also stress the knee joint and connective tissue.

- Turning or "torquing" your hips or letting them drop to one side to get a deeper lunge, which can stress your spine and cause alignment problems with your pelvis.

- Only focusing on the working leg; you should be aware of the alignment of the stabilizing leg as well.

- Causing lower back problems by not paying special attention to your posture as you go down into a squat or lunge; don't arch your back to get deeper.

- Over-rotating feet on turned-out exercises like the plié, which can place a great deal of stress on hip and knee joints.

- "Bouncing" at the end—or bottom—of a squat or lunge, which can cause painful groin pulls.

The Moves

21a

21b

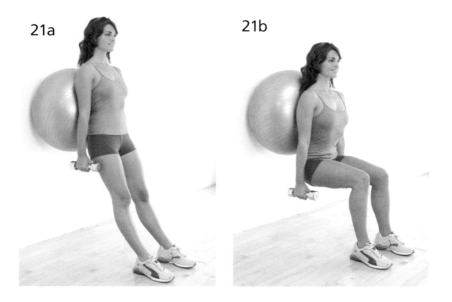

21. Wall ball squat (B): Place a stability ball between a wall and your back. Holding a dumbbell in each hand, arms at sides, palms in, and abdominals pulled in, walk feet forward 1–2 feet so that your torso can lean comfortably against the ball. Draw shoulder blades together and down to stabilize upper back; keep chest lifted and shoulders relaxed (a). Bend knees and lower hips until thighs are parallel to the floor and knees are bent at 90 degrees; don't let hips press back as you lower (b). Straighten legs to starting position without locking knees and repeat.

Weight: 5–12 pounds.

Strengthens buttocks, quadriceps, and hamstrings; upper hips and inner thighs work as stabilizers.

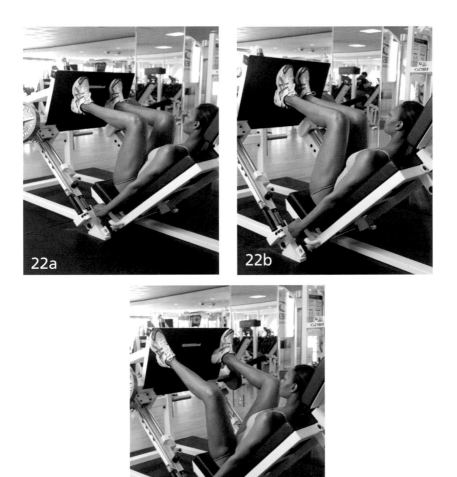

22. 3-position leg press (B, I, A): Sit on a leg-press machine with the seat back adjusted to 45 degrees. Place feet hip-width apart in center of foot plate with knees bent; hold handles for support. Contract abdominals; spine is supported against back pad. Release machine locks and straighten legs, keeping knees and feet aligned. Bend knees toward chest until they align with hips (a). Straighten legs and repeat for specified number of reps. Reposition legs with feet only slightly apart and repeat the same movement for the recommended amount of reps (b). Last, place feet near the top of the foot plate with toes and knees turned out. Bend knees, keeping toes and knees aligned, until thighs align with hips (c). Straighten legs and repeat for specified number of reps.

Weight: 0–90 pounds of added weight on each side.

Strengthens buttocks, quadriceps, and hamstrings; upper hips and inner thighs work as stabilizers.

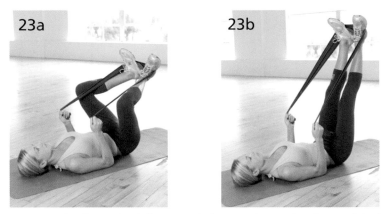

23. Froggies (B, I, A): Lie faceup and place a resistance band around the balls of your feet; then bend knees in toward chest, heels together with toes turned out. Hold one end of the band in each hand, elbows on the floor and bent, palms facing in and knuckles pointing upward. Contract your abdominals, drawing hips and tailbone down toward the floor to stabilize your position (a). Keep heels together and inhale, then exhale and press legs out until they're straight and as low to the floor as you can get them while maintaining a stable pelvis (b). Inhale, bending legs back to starting position and repeat.

Weight: Medium to heavy resistance.

Strengthens quadriceps, inner thighs, buttocks, hamstrings, and hip rotators; abdominals and spine extensors work as stabilizers.

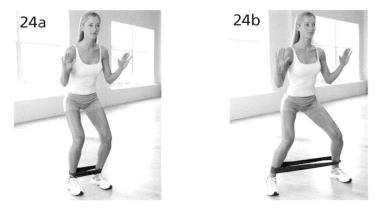

24. Lateral shuffle (B, I, A): Tie a resistance band around your legs at mid-shin level, so you have tension on upper hips when feet are hip-width apart. Bend elbows close to torso and in front of you, contract abs, and draw shoulder blades down and together to keep torso erect. Bend knees into a quarter-squat (a). Maintaining the squat position, step sideways to the left with left foot (b). Still squatting, bring right foot toward left while maintaining the distance between feet and the tension on band. Continue to squat for reps to the left; then return to the right as you shuffle, pressing out against band to keep knees from collapsing inward.

Weight: Light to medium resistance.

Strengthens upper hips, inner thighs, quadriceps, hamstrings, and buttocks; abdominals and spine extensors work as stabilizers.

training for tighter thighs

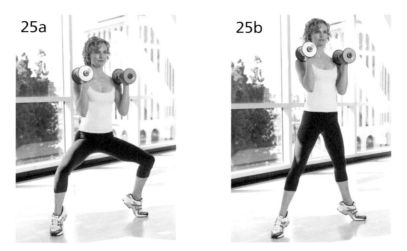

25. Plié/relevé (I–A): Hold a dumbbell on each shoulder with elbows bent. Stand with feet slightly more than hip-width apart, turning toes and knees out comfortably. Pull abdominals in so that tailbone points down toward the floor with chest lifted and shoulders relaxed. Keeping torso erect, bend knees to lower hips toward the floor in a plié, but only as far as possible without tucking tailbone under or arching back. Maintain this position and rise up onto the balls of your feet (a). Stay lifted and straighten legs (b). Lower heels to the floor and repeat.

Weight: 5–8 pounds in each hand.

Strengthens quadriceps, inner thighs, buttocks, hamstrings, and calves.

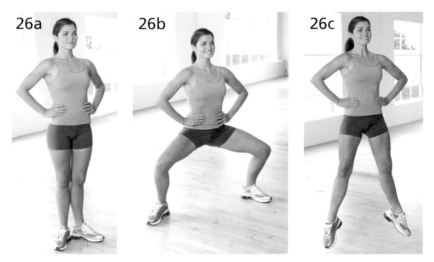

26. Plié jump and drag (I–A): Stand with heels together, toes and knees turned out comfortably, and hands on hips. Pull abdominals in so that tailbone points down toward the floor; chest is lifted, and shoulders are relaxed (a). Keeping torso erect, step out to the left and bend knees into a plié, lowering hips to the floor only as far as possible without tucking tailbone under or arching back (b). Push off both feet, straightening legs as you jump up in the air, lengthening legs and pointing toes (c). Land in plié with bent knees. As you straighten legs, drag left foot back to meet the right one, heels together in starting position. Repeat, this time stepping out to the right. Continue to alternate for the specified number of reps.

Strengthens quadriceps, inner thighs, upper hips, buttocks, hamstrings, and calves.

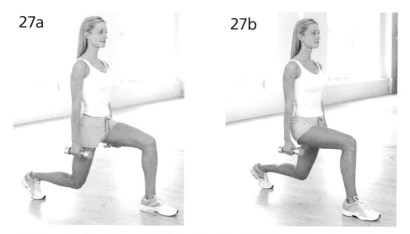

27. Front-to-back lunge (I–A): Holding dumbbells in each hand, arms hanging down at sides, and palms facing in, stand with feet hip-width apart and legs straight, but not locked. Contract abdominals so that spine is neutral, and squeeze shoulder blades together and down. Take a step forward with one foot and bend knees, lowering hips toward the floor until front knee is bent at 90 degrees and back knee is pointing down with back heel lifted (a). Straighten legs and step backward with the same leg, lowering hips into a lunge (b). Straighten legs and repeat both front and back lunges on the same side, then switch legs.

Strengthens buttocks, quadriceps, hamstrings, and calves; upper hips and inner thighs work as stabilizers.

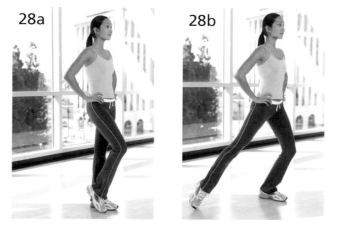

28. Skate lunge (I–A): Standing with hands on hips and feet together, shift weight to left foot so that only toes of right foot touch the ground and right knee is bent (a). Contract abs to maintain a tall, neutral spine, then bend left knee as you press right foot diagonally out to right side, toes still touching the ground (b). Drag toes of right foot back to starting position, straightening left knee. Do all reps on one side, then switch legs and repeat on the opposite side to complete one set.

Strengthens quadriceps, hamstrings, buttocks, upper hips, and inner thighs.

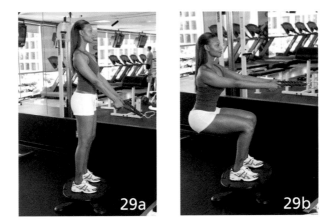

29. Balanced low cable squat (I–A): Attach a rope to a low-cable-pulley machine. Face the machine and grasp one end of the rope in each hand, then stand on a stability tool (such as a Reebok Core Board) with feet hip-width apart and find your balance. Extend arms toward cable, keeping shoulder blades down and squeezed together and neck aligned with spine (a). Bend both knees, sitting down and back into a squat, lowering hips until thighs are parallel to the floor, knees aligned with toes (b). Pause, holding squat for a count, then straighten legs to standing position without locking knees and repeat.

Weight: 20–50 pounds.

Strengthens quadriceps, hamstrings, and buttocks; upper hips, inner thighs, abdominals, and spine extensors work as stabilizers.

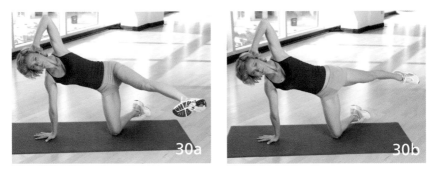

30. Kneeling side plank with leg sweeps (A): Kneel on your right knee and extend your left leg out to the side on the floor. Place right hand on the floor, aligning wrist under right shoulder, arm straight but not locked, and place left hand behind head with elbow bent. Contract abdominals, bringing spine to a neutral position, then lift left leg up to hip height, foot flexed so that body forms a straight line from shoulders to heel. Maintain torso position and bring left leg as far forward as you can without changing alignment (a). Then sweep leg back behind you, still at hip height, while pointing toe and keeping hips squared and stacked in order to complete one rep (b). Continue forward and back sweep for the specified number of reps, then switch sides and repeat to complete one set.

Strengthens upper hips, inner thighs, buttocks, quadriceps, and hamstrings; abdominals and spine extensors work as stabilizers.

Ultimate Word

Do you want to know a secret for sleek, superdefined legs? According to Philip Dozois, a certified trainer and co-owner of Breakthru Fitness in Pasadena, California, it's stretching. "[It] can help you get stronger," he confirms. "You'll improve your range of motion, and stretching may enhance recovery. It increases blood flow to your muscles, delivering fresh nutrients and flushing out waste products."

For maximum muscle tone, he recommends doing quadriceps stretches between sets of quad moves, as well as after your workout. "The quadriceps tend to get tight, especially if you spend a lot of time sitting during the day," Dozois explains. "If you don't stretch them, you'll be setting yourself up for possible knee problems and muscle imbalance."

The same thing applies to your hamstrings: Stretch them out between sets of hamstring exercises. These muscles can tighten if you run, walk, or cycle on level ground (instead of hills) and don't fully extend your legs and hips regularly.

Now that you have a full complement of programs to help you get in shape from the waist down, we're going to move on and start working your upper body, beginning in the next chapter.

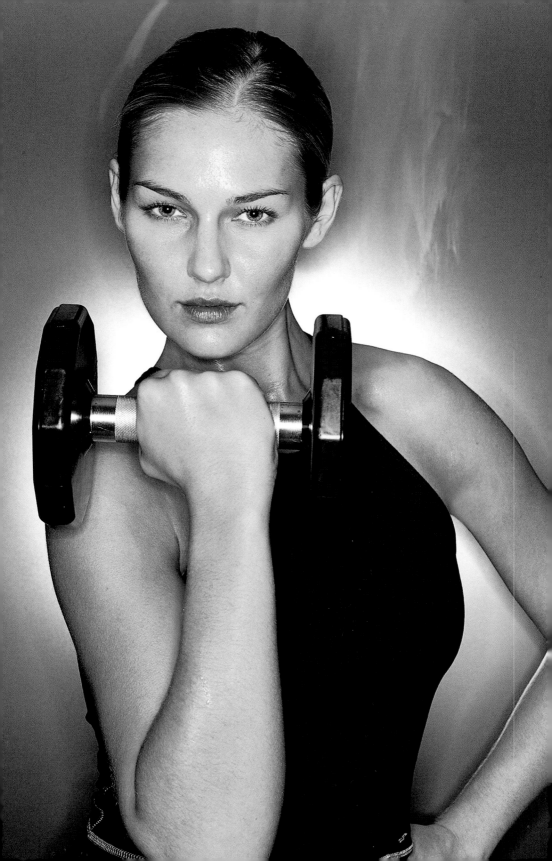

chapter 5

a beautiful upper body

It's possible get so fixated on traditional trouble spots such as the butt or thighs that you neglect your upper body. After all, your arms are often undercover in the long-sleeved shirts, jackets, and sweaters that you wear to work. Wouldn't you like to show them off in a strapless dress at night or a swimsuit in summer? In addition, you'll want to head off those flabby upper arms that can develop from inactivity as you age. Upper-body work will also help improve your posture, and give you strength for everyday activities.

This Chapter's To-Do List

In these pages you'll learn:

- The truth about upper body workouts
- The ten best moves for toning your back, shoulders, and arms
- Four-week training programs for beginning, intermediate, and advanced exercisers
- What to avoid when working your upper body muscles

Do You Know the Truth about Upper-Body Training?

Amazing arms and a strong back can be yours if you go about it in the right way. Answer "true" or "false" to the following questions to see if you have the right attitude about upper-body workouts.

1. You shouldn't weight-train your upper body because women don't look feminine with bulky arms.

False. Don't worry about getting big arms. "Women just don't have enough testosterone to build large amounts of muscle," says Keli Roberts, a spokeswoman for the American Council on Exercise and group fitness manager at Equinox Fitness Club in Pasadena, California. "It's actually very difficult for women to get big." Getting rid of arm flab is a two-part process: You need to reduce the fat that sits on top by burning more calories than you eat, and at the same time you need to tone the muscles underneath.

2. If you're a runner, you don't need to worry about your upper body.

False. Strong upper bodies aren't just for tennis and volleyball players. "I've trained runners whose [race] times improved dramatically after they started training their upper bodies," says Irene McCormick, the coordinator of recreation, fitness, and wellness programs at the Des Moines Area Community Colleges in Iowa.

3. If you're "bottom heavy," you're better off spending your time toning below your waist than above it.

False. "When we've got a body part we don't like, we tend to train it mercilessly," says Phil Dozois, co-owner of Breakthru Fitness in Pasadena, California. "People don't realize that besides dropping body fat, the best way to make any area of your body look smaller is to make other parts look a little bigger and more shapely. If you have an apple- or pear-shaped body, shapely shoulders will balance the hips and will make them look smaller," he explains. Besides, no matter what shape you want to achieve, you'll need to do full-body strength training rather than concentrating on only one area.

4. Exercising your back can make you look like a linebacker.

False. Review our response to the first myth, because everything we said about your shoulders applies equally to your back. If you're looking for an easy way to change your appearance, develop this part of your body. A beautiful V-shaped back can minimize your waist and lower body, and strength in this area improves your posture and encourages you to stand taller. In everyday life, you may tend to perform forward moves with your arms and the front portion of your upper body; working the opposing muscle groups prevents imbalances that can cause injury.

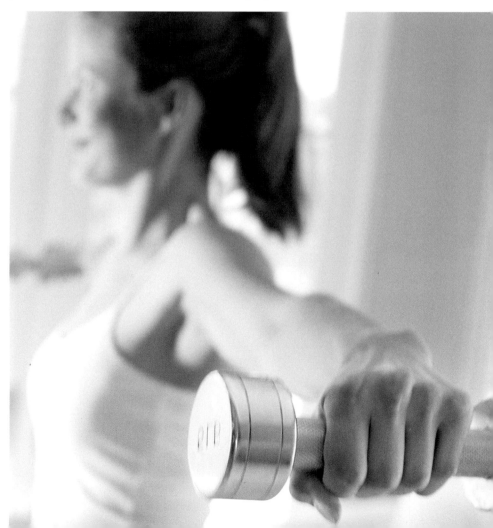

Q.   **When and how should you stretch?**

A.   You can stretch anytime you feel like it, or you can do so in conjunction with other workouts. Just remember: Stretch *after* any type of physical activity—cardio, strength training, or sports. Muscles are warmer and more pliable then, making it easier to lengthen them. According to Wayne Westcott, Ph.D., fitness research director of the South Shore YMCA in Quincy, Massachusetts, vigorous stretching before exercise, when muscles are cold and less pliable, will produce less benefit and may leave tendons more susceptible to injury. A good rule of thumb is to start your workout with a five-minute cardio warm-up, stretch gently, and follow your usual routine. Then do more serious stretching after you're finished.

Here are a few tips to keep in mind:

- Don't bounce. Using momentum to increase your stretch can activate the body's protective reflex, causing the muscles to contract instead of stretch, which can lead to small tears.

- Don't stretch to the point of pain. While you may experience a little discomfort in an area that's tight, actual pain is your body's way of letting you know that something's wrong.

- Don't forget to breathe. Not only is oxygen exchange necessary for the muscle to respond to a stretch in a beneficial way, but holding your breath may temporarily increase blood pressure. Focus on inhaling as you get into position for the stretch, and exhaling as you move deeper into it. And keep your breathing slow and regular.

The Workouts

Although there are many individual muscles in your upper body, you don't have to worry about exercising each one individually. The three levels of workouts in this chapter—beginning, intermediate, and advanced—incorporate moves that work several muscles at a time so that you get the best results.

You'll know which one of the three programs you should start with by taking our fitness test. (If you haven't completed it yet, go back and do so.) Each has variations in the moves you'll perform (labeled B, I, and A); the number of sets and reps you'll do; and the amount of weight you'll use (if applicable).

We've given you guidelines to follow for each of the three levels, so read them and make sure that you understand the instructions before beginning. Every exercise is numbered, which lets you know where to find the description of how to do it and see it demonstrated in the corresponding photographs. Always warm up with five minutes of light cardio activity, and complete your workout by stretching the muscles worked, holding each stretch for 30 seconds without bouncing.

Each workout is a progressive four-week program that you can do either at home or in the gym. You'll move from beginner to intermediate to advanced after completing each four-week program, or when you're ready to go on to the next level. Repeat the lower-level regimens if your form is poor, you don't feel that you've mastered the moves, or you can't complete the recommended sets or reps with the suggested weight. Even if you are advanced, you might find it beneficial to go back and perform a beginner exercise for variety and to reestablish your form.

The moves in this chapter target your entire upper body: the middle and upper back, shoulders, chest, and arms. Let's take a look at the muscles involved in the workouts, and how they all fit together.

Your main upper-back muscles are the trapezius and rhomboids. The trapezius attaches to the base of your skull, the midback vertebrae, and both ends of your collarbone. The top part assists in overhead pushing, the middle pulls your shoulder blades together, and the lower region draws your arms toward your body. The rhomboids, located between your shoulder blades, stabilize your upper back and shoulders.

The latissimus dorsi (or *lat*), the largest muscle in the upper body, covers the lower and middle portions of the back, originating on the spine and the top of the hip bone and attaching to the upper arm. The lat is responsible for downward movements of the upper arm (such as pulling your elbows down and in toward your waist), pulling your arms behind you, and helping with inward rotation of the shoulder. The teres major, a small muscle that originates on the inside lower edge of the shoulder blade and attaches on the upper-arm bone (the humerus), performs these same movements.

The deltoids—your shoulder muscles—consist of three "heads," and while each has different origins, they all attach on your upper arm. The anterior head originates at your collarbone and moves your arm up and forward, as well as rotating it inward. The posterior head attaches to your shoulder blade and moves your arm to the rear, as well as rotating it outward. The lateral head (which is located between the other two) primarily works to lift your arm to the side and assists the anterior and posterior heads in their movements. Your rotator-cuff muscles—the supraspinatus, infraspinatus, teres minor, and subscapularis—stabilize your shoulder joint.

The main chest muscle is the pectoralis major, a large fan-shaped muscle that has multiple attachments: One portion fastens to the middle and inner parts of your collarbone, working with the anterior deltoid to move your arms forward and upward and rotate them inward. The other part attaches to your breastbone (the sternum) and upper six ribs, and is stimulated only in downward and forward movements of the arms. Both of these portions come together near the top of your upper-arm bones.

The serratus anterior (located on either side of your rib cage) and the pectorals minor (a small muscle that's deep under the pectoralis major) help stabilize your shoulder blades when your arms move forward.

There are two primary muscles on the front of your upper arm: the biceps brachii and the brachialis. Both help flex your elbow and rotate your forearm so that your palms can face up or down. The biceps brachii has two heads—one long, one short—that cross your shoulder joint at different places and attach onto the shoulder blade, then insert together on your forearm, just below the elbow joint. The brachialis, the larger of the two muscles and your strongest elbow flexor, lies deep beneath the biceps brachii, crossing your elbow joint.

The triceps, on the rear of your upper arm, is one muscle comprising three sections that are joined together in a common tendon below the elbow. Together the lateral, medial, and long heads extend your elbow to straighten your arm. Both the lateral and medial heads originate on the upper-arm bone and the long head crosses the shoulder joint, attaching on the shoulder blade.

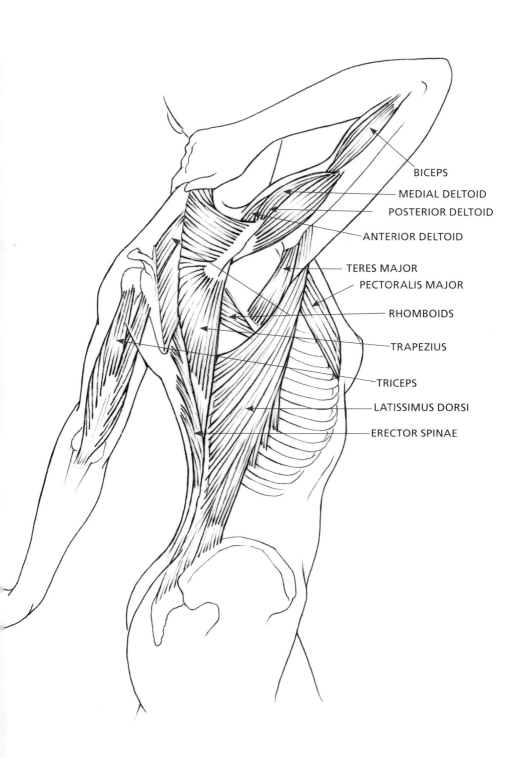

BICEPS

MEDIAL DELTOID

POSTERIOR DELTOID

ANTERIOR DELTOID

TERES MAJOR

PECTORALIS MAJOR

RHOMBOIDS

TRAPEZIUS

TRICEPS

LATISSIMUS DORSI

ERECTOR SPINAE

Beginners

Guidelines: Do these exercises (see page 97 for "The Moves") twice a week with at least 1 day of rest in between workouts. Perform the suggested number of reps for each move, and rest 45–60 seconds between sets. However, when you see the superset, do the 2 exercises grouped together consecutively, without resting between them; rest 45–60 seconds between supersets.

Week One

Exercise	Sets	Reps
31. Close grip lat pull-down	1–2	8–12
35. Standing cable chest fly	1–2	8–12
32. High cable press-down	1–2	8–12
33. Biceps curl	1–2	8–12

Week Two

Exercise	Sets	Reps
31. Close grip lat pull-down	2	8–12
35. Standing cable chest fly	2	8–12
32. High cable press-down	2	8–12
33. Biceps curl	2	8–12

Week Three

Exercise	Sets	Reps
31. Close grip lat pull-down	2	10–12
33. Biceps curl	2	10–12
34. Overhead press	2	8–12
35. Standing cable chest fly	2	10–12
32. High cable press-down	2	10–15

Exercise		Sets	Reps
Superset:	*31. Close grip lat pull-down*	2	10–12
	34. Overhead press	2	10–12
35. Standing cable chest fly		2	10–12
Superset:	*33. Biceps curl*	2	10–15
	32. High cable press-down	2	10–15

Her Ultimate Turning Point

Pictures taken at her graduation from cosmetology school finally made Stacie Lafler of Ohio realize that she needed to get her weight under control. "I didn't recognize myself, and I could see that my size-14 clothes were tight on me," she says. Stacie first focused on following a cardio regimen and ran up to ten miles a day, but only lost five pounds after six months. She shared her frustration with one of her clients, a personal trainer, who told Stacie that she was doing too much cardio and needed to weight-train in order to build muscle. So she started weight training at the gym twice a week to complement her existing workouts, which she cut to three or four miles a session.

Just a few weeks later, Stacie felt better than she had in years. "The muscle I built helped me lose three to five pounds a month," she says. Later, when she wanted to lose some postpartum weight, Stacie added boxing, jumping rope, and elliptical training (all good upper-body toners) to her routine.

Her Best Tip: Think of exercising and eating right as a lifelong commitment. "I wouldn't have it any other way," she says. "I've never been this fit in my whole life, and it feels incredible."

Intermediate

Guidelines: Do these exercises (see page 97 for "The Moves") 2–3 times a week with a day of rest in between workouts. Perform the suggested number of reps for each move, and rest 45–60 seconds between sets. However, where you see the superset, do the 2 exercises grouped together consecutively without resting between them; rest 45–60 seconds between supersets.

Week One

Exercise	Sets	Reps
31. Close grip lat pull-down	2–3	8–12
40. Reciprocal ball chest press	2–3	8–12
34. Overhead press	2–3	8–12
36. Seated bent-over rear fly	2–3	8–12
33. Biceps curl	2–3	10–12
32. High cable press-down	2–3	10–12

Week Two

Exercise	Sets	Reps
37. Seated cable high row	2–3	8–12
35. Standing cable chest fly	2–3	8–12
39. Shoulder fan	2–3	5–6
Superset: *33. Biceps curl*	2–3	10–15
38. Bent-over triceps kickback	2–3	10–15

Week Three

Exercise	Sets	Reps
Superset: *31. Close grip lat pull-down*	2–3	10–12
33. Biceps curl	2–3	10–12

Exercise		Sets	Reps
Superset:	40. Reciprocal ball chest press	2–3	8–12
	32. High cable press-down	2–3	10–12
Superset:	34. Overhead press	2–3	10–12
	36. Seated bent-over fly	2–3	8–12

Week Four

Choose from the following programs each session:

Exercise		Sets	Reps
Workout 1			
Superset:	31. Close grip lat pull-down	2–3	10–12
	33. Biceps curl	2–3	10–12
Superset:	40. Reciprocal ball chest press	2–3	8–12
	32. High cable press-down	2–3	10–12
Superset:	34. Overhead press	2–3	10–12
	36. Seated bent-over rear fly	2–3	8–12
Workout 2			
37. Seated cable high row		2–3	10–12
34. Overhead press		2–3	10–12
40. Reciprocal ball chest press		2–3	8–12
32. High cable press-down		2–3	10–15
39. Shoulder fan		2–3	5–6
33. Biceps curl		2–3	10–12
Workout 3			
Superset:	31. Close grip lat pull-down	2–3	8–12
	37. Seated cable high row	2–3	8–12
Superset:	40. Reciprocal ball chest press	2–3	8–12
	35. Standing cable chest fly	2–3	8–12
Superset:	34. Overhead press	2–3	8–12
	36. Seated bent-over fly	2–3	8–12
Superset:	32. High cable press-down	2–3	8–12
	38. Bent-over triceps kickbacks	2–3	8–12

Advanced

Guidelines: Do these exercises (see page 97 for "The Moves") 2–3 times a week with a day of rest in between workouts. Perform the suggested number of reps for each move, and rest 45–60 seconds between sets. However, where you see the superset, do the 2 exercises grouped together consecutively without pausing between them; rest 45–60 seconds between supersets.

Week One

Exercise	Sets	Reps
31. Close grip lat pull-down	2–3	8–12
40. Reciprocal ball chest press	2–3	8–12
35. Standing cable chest fly	2–3	10–12
34. Overhead press	2–3	10–12
36. Seated bent-over rear fly	2–3	8–12
33. Biceps curl	2–3	10–15
32. High cable press-down	2–3	10–15
38. Bent-over triceps kickback	2–3	8–12

Week Two

Exercise	Sets	Reps
37. Seated cable high row	2–3	8–12
31. Close grip lat pull-down	2–3	8–12
35. Standing cable chest fly	2–3	10–12
40. Reciprocal ball chest press	2–3	8–12
39. Shoulder fan	2–3	5–6
34. Overhead press	2–3	10–12
Superset: *33. Biceps curl*	2–3	10–15
38. Bent-over triceps kickback	2–3	10–15

Week Three

Exercise		Sets	Reps
Superset:	31. Close grip lat pull-down	2–3	10–12
	33. Biceps curl	2–3	10–12
Superset:	40. Reciprocal ball chest press	2–3	8–12
	32. High cable press-down	2–3	10–12
38. Bent over triceps kickback		2–3	10–12
Superset:	34. Overhead press	2–3	10–12
	36. Seated bent-over rear fly	2–3	8–12
Superset:	37. Seated cable high row	2–3	8–12
	39. Shoulder fan	2–3	5–6

Week Four

Choose from the following programs for each session:

Exercise		Sets	Reps
Workout 1			
Superset:	31. Close grip lat pull-down	2–3	10–12
	33. Biceps curl	2–3	10–12
Superset:	40. Reciprocal ball chest press	2–3	10–12
	32. High cable press-down	2–3	10–15
38. Bent over triceps kickback		2–3	10–15
Superset:	34. Overhead press	2–3	10–12
	36. Seated bent-over fly	2–3	10–12
Superset:	37. Seated cable high row	2–3	8–12
	39. Shoulder fan	2–3	5–6
Workout 2			
37. Seated cable high row		2–3	10–12
34. Overhead press		2–3	10–12
40. Reciprocal ball chest press		2–3	8–12
32. High cable press-down		2–3	10–15
39. Shoulder fan		2–3	5–6

Exercise	Sets	Reps
36. Seated bent-over fly	2–3	8–12
33. Biceps curl	2–3	10–15

Workout 3

		Sets	Reps
Superset:	*31. Close grip lat pull-down*	2–3	8–12
	37. Seated cable high row	2–3	8–12
Superset:	*40. Reciprocal ball chest press*	2–3	8–12
	35. Standing cable chest fly	2–3	8–12
Superset:	*34. Overhead press*	2–3	8–12
	36. Seated bent over fly	2–3	8–12
39. Shoulder fan		2–3	8–12
33. Biceps curl		2–3	8–15
Superset:	*32. High cable press-down*	2–3	8–12
	38. Bent-over triceps kickbacks	2–3	8–12

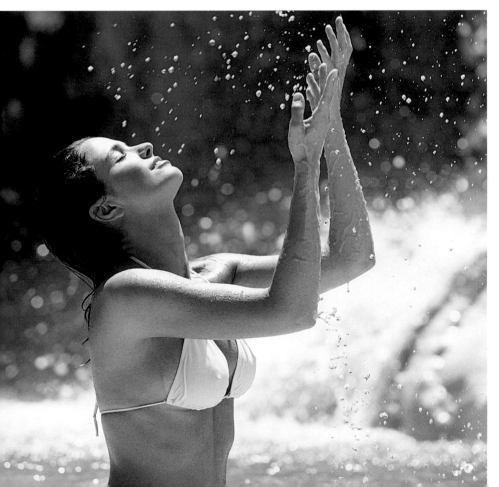

The Moves

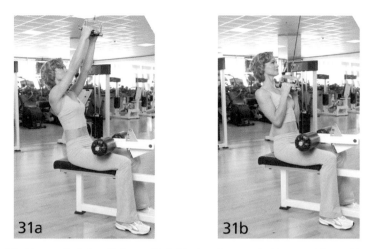

31a   31b

31. Close grip lat pull-down (B, I, A): Attach an angled bar to a high-cable pulley, then grasp the bar, sit down, and position thighs under pads with feet flat on the floor, knees bent and in line with ankles. Lean entire torso slightly back from hips so the bar is above breastbone with arms straight, wrists neutral, and palms facing in. Contract abdominals, keep chest lifted, and draw shoulder blades down and together (a). Bend elbows down and back toward waist, bringing the bar down toward your upper chest as you lift chest up toward the bar (b). Pause and straighten arms to starting position and repeat.

Weight: 30–75 pounds.
Strengthens upper and middle back and rear of shoulders.

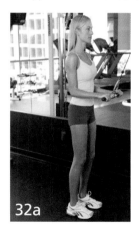 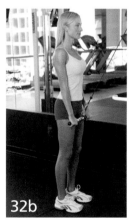

32a   32b

32. High cable press-down (B, I, A): Attach a straight bar to a high-cable pulley. Stand facing the weight stack with feet hip-width apart and knees slightly bent. Grasp bar with an overhand grip, hands shoulder-width apart. Contract abdominals to bring spine into a neutral position, lift chest, and draw shoulder blades together and down. Bend elbows, aligning them under shoulders with upper arms close to torso, forearms parallel, and wrists straight (a). Keep torso erect and straighten arms, pressing bar down toward thighs while keeping wrists straight (b). Pause, then slowly bend elbows to starting position without changing shoulder or elbow alignment, and repeat.

Weight: 20–50 pounds.
Strengthens triceps.

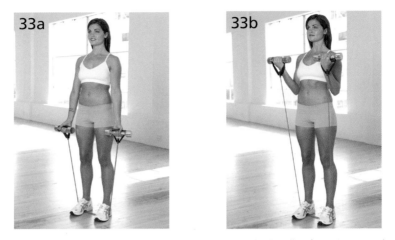

33. Biceps curl (B, I, A): Holding a dumbbell and the handle of a resistance tube in each hand, stand on the tube with feet hip-width apart, legs straight but not locked. Let arms hang at sides of thighs, elbows aligned under shoulders, palms facing forward. Pull abs in, keeping chest lifted and shoulders relaxed (a). Maintain elbow position and keep shoulders motionless as you bend elbows and bring dumbbells up toward shoulders with wrists straight, resisting the additional tension of the tube (b). Slowly straighten arms without locking elbows and repeat.

Weight: 5- to 8-pound dumbbells, and a light- to medium-resistance tube. Strengthens biceps.

34. Overhead press (B, I, A): Stand with feet hip-width apart, legs straight but not locked. Hold a dumbbell in each hand at shoulder height with elbows pointing toward the floor, forearms parallel to each other, wrists straight, and palms facing forward. Contract abdominals to bring spine into a neutral position with chest lifted and shoulders relaxed (a). Draw shoulder blades together and down, then straighten arms overhead, rotating palms to face each other by the top of the lift without locking elbows or torquing wrists (b). Bend elbows and lower dumbbells, rotating palms forward to starting position, and repeat.

Weight: 5–10 pounds.
Strengthens upper back and front and middle of shoulders.

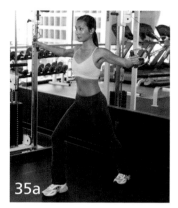
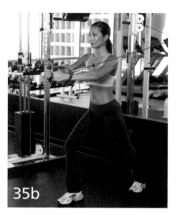

35. Standing cable chest fly (B, I, A): Attach single handles to each upper cable in a cable cage, then grasp a handle in each hand with an overhand grip. Stand centered and just behind both cables in a staggered stance, leaning slightly forward from your ankles. Contract abdominals to bring spine into a neutral position, and squeeze shoulder blades together and down. Extend arms out at shoulder height and in line with cables with elbows lifted and bent in a soft arc, palms facing in, and wrists neutral (a). Maintaining elbow arc, press handles together in front at midchest height until knuckles almost touch (b). Open arms to starting position without rocking, and repeat.

Weight: 10–30 pounds on each cable.

Strengthens chest and front of shoulder.

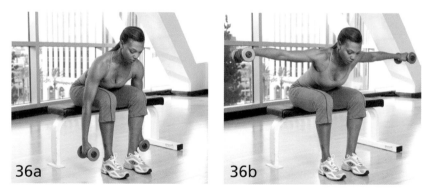

36. Seated bent-over rear fly (I–A): Sit on a bench with feet hip-width apart, knees bent and aligned over ankles. Hold a dumbbell in each hand, arms at sides. Bend forward from hips so that torso hovers over thighs and back is straight. Let arms hang straight down and in line with shoulders, elbows in a slight arc, palms facing in, and wrists straight. Draw shoulder blades down and together, moving ears away from shoulders while keeping head and neck aligned with spine (a). Maintain position and contract upper-back muscles to lift arms up and out to the sides, keeping wrists neutral, until elbows are even with shoulders (b). Pause, then slowly lower to starting position and repeat.

Weight: 3–8 pounds.

Strengthens rear of shoulders and upper back; abdominals and spine extensors work as stabilizers.

a beautiful upper body

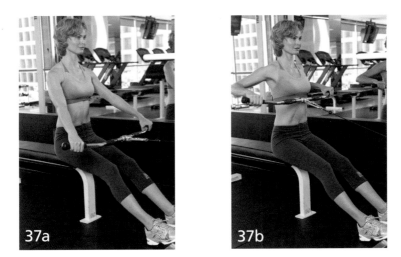

37. Seated cable high row (I–A): Attach a long bar to a low-cable pulley machine, then sit erect on a bench with feet hip-width apart on the support plate or bar, knees slightly bent, and toes pointing up. Bend forward from hips and grasp bar with an overhand grip wider than shoulder width, then sit erect with arms extended and palms down. Contract abs to bring spine into neutral position, drawing shoulder blades down and together (a). Maintain position and bend elbows out and back until bar just touches upper rib cage, elbows even with shoulders (b). Straighten arms to starting position without collapsing torso and repeat.

Weight: 20–50 pounds.

Strengthens upper back and rear of shoulders.

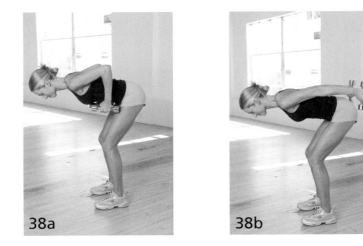

38. Bent-over triceps kickback (I–A): Standing with feet hip-width apart and a dumbbell in each hand, bend knees and hinge forward from hips until back is parallel to the floor. Bend elbows so that they're close to torso with palms facing in, upper arms stable, and knuckles pointing down toward the floor. Pull in abs to stabilize spine (a). Maintain position and straighten arms behind you until elbows are fully extended, but not locked (b). Pause, then bend elbows to starting position and repeat.

Weight: 3–8 pounds.

Strengthens triceps.

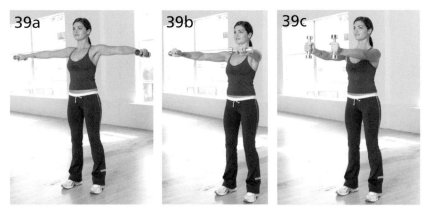

39. Shoulder fan (I–A): Hold a dumbbell in each hand with arms hanging at sides and palms facing in. Stand with feet hip-width apart, knees slightly bent, and weight balanced evenly between toes and heels. Contract abs to bring spine into a neutral position with chest lifted, shoulders relaxed, neck long, and chin level. Maintain a slight arc in elbows and lift arms up and out to sides, up to shoulder height, with palms down and wrists straight (a). Lower arms to starting position, then lift them up to a 45-degree angle to shoulder height (b). Lower, and then lift arms up in front of you, with palms facing in (c). Lower to complete one rep, and then repeat the "fan."

Weight: 3–5 pounds.

Strengthens front and middle shoulder; upper back muscles work as stabilizers.

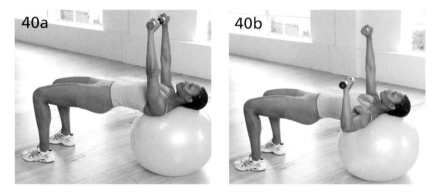

40. Reciprocal ball chest press (I–A): Sitting on a stability ball with a dumbbell in each hand, walk feet forward until just head, neck, and upper back are supported on the ball. Keep knees bent and aligned over ankles, with feet flat on the floor. Raise arms above midchest, palms facing forward, and wrists straight. Contract abdominals to bring spine into a neutral position; squeeze shoulder blades together and down to stabilize upper back on the ball and tighten buttocks to keep hips lifted (a). Bend left elbow, lowering dumbbell down and out to the side of chest until elbow is bent to 90 degrees and aligns with shoulder, wrist aligned over elbow (b). Straighten arm, pushing dumbbell up to start position as you lower right dumbbell at the same time to complete one rep. Continue to alternate arms for the specified number of reps while keeping stable on the ball.

Weight: 5–15 pounds.

Strengthens chest, front of shoulders, and triceps.

a beautiful upper body

Ultimate Word

To get the most from your upper-body moves, pay close attention to your posture, advises Jessica Perry, a certified trainer at Chelsea Piers in New York City. To target your muscles correctly, you need to be impeccable about proper alignment, she explains. Stay aware of your position and focus on how your body is moving in every rep.

The upper body programs in this chapter were the final pieces for working individual muscle groups. In the next chapter, we're going to put them all together for your Ultimate Body!

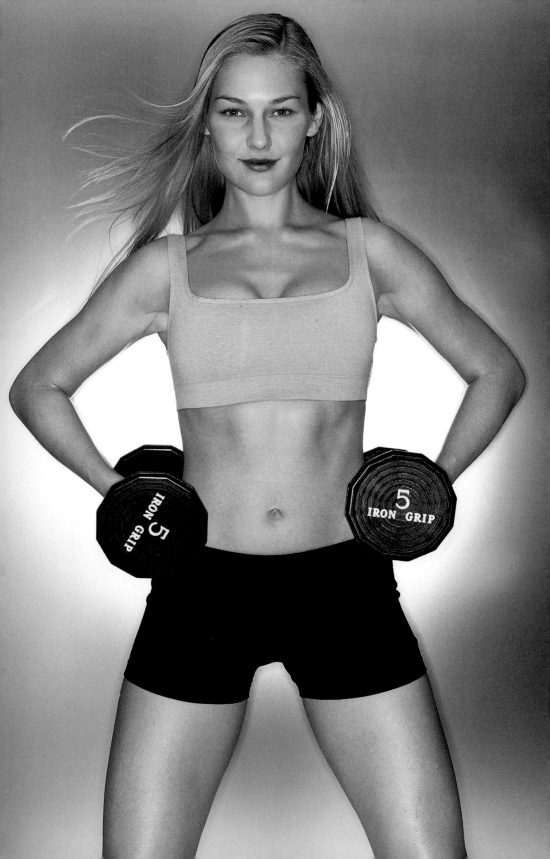

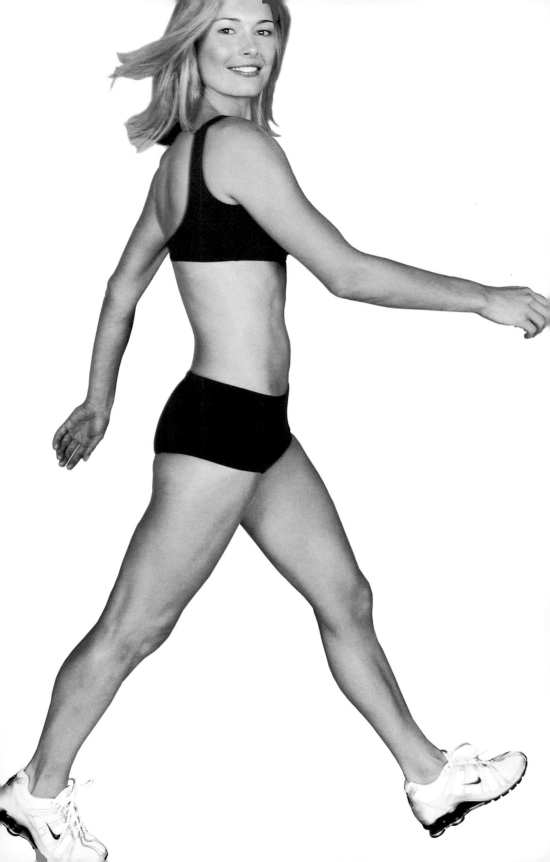

chapter 6

your total-body program

In the previous four chapters, you learned individual programs for working your abs, butt and hips, thighs, and upper body. Now you're going to put them all together in a program that will get you on the fast track to an energized, strong, healthy self—your Ultimate Body.

This Chapter's To-Do List

In the following pages, you'll learn:

- Why these workouts are so effective
- How to use moves from the previous chapters to strengthen and tone your total body
- Four-week training programs for beginning, intermediate, and advanced exercisers
- Tips for making the most of your regimen

Program Design

As with the exercises for individual body parts, this chapter also has three levels of total-body workouts: beginning, intermediate, and advanced. Each one is a four-week progressive strength-training plan that works your entire body in each session. There are variations in the moves you'll perform (found in the individual body-part chapters); the number of sets and reps you'll do; and the amount of weight you'll use (if applicable).

The beginner workouts are based on building a solid foundation, which will fine-tune your form so that you can strengthen muscles that are typically weak and imbalanced and progress with ease. Most of the exercises for the beginning level use multiple muscles and are performed in a stable, secure position so that you can learn to add weight effectively and improve your overall coordination safely. You should complete each session of the beginner's program in about 20 minutes.

Built into your program is a blend of alternating upper- and lower-body exercises so that you can continue to exercise without too much fatigue. You'll perform moves such as the seated bent-over rear fly, which strengthens your deepest mid-back muscles and increases muscular endurance that's crucial for posture and for keeping you upright with less effort. In contrast, the lateral shuffle will strengthen your upper hips and quadriceps to protect your knees. The fourth week, you'll add a superset to prepare you to move beyond the beginner's plan.

The intermediate program will take you to the next level of training, where you'll complete more exercises and sets, and the overall workout will be more challenging. These sessions should take about 30 to 35 minutes to complete.

You'll still perform some of the same exercises that are included in the beginner's program; however, they'll be in a different sequence. You'll start with techniques like supersets and prefatigue training in the first week, plus you'll typically do more than one exercise in a row per body part. This level includes more balance and core challenges, and adds weight to basic exercises (such as holding a dumbbell while you crunch). However, you'll still do foundation exercises to help you maintain overall alignment and muscle balance.

The advanced program, which will take you between 35 and 45 minutes to complete, is designed to further add definition and shape to your muscles by manipulating the order in which you do the exercises. By the time you reach these workouts, your body will be able to handle consistent training without the amount of rest between sets that you need in the lower-level programs. The advanced regimen introduces more techniques (such as tri-sets), along with multiple supersets to really challenge your strength and endurance.

Foundation exercises such as the three-position leg press and close-grip lat pull-down are combined with those that work the muscles stabilizing your posture and balance. You'll still be doing many of the moves from the two previous programs, with the additional challenge of the multiple supersets and tri-sets that put this program a step above the rest.

Training Techniques

Certain training techniques can take your resistance program to the next level, promoting greater muscle gain, jolting your metabolism, pushing you past a plateau, supercharging your motivation, and so much more. These are called "high-intensity training techniques." Don't let the name intimidate you, because even if you're a beginner, they can still add challenge to your workouts, particularly when simply upping the amount of weight you're lifting isn't the best option.

The four-week, multilevel plans in this chapter were designed with some of these techniques in mind (and for even more advanced training techniques, see Chapter 11). There's not only a sequential logic to the exercise selection for each workout level, but there's also a specific order built into the programs over the four weeks that will help you exercise efficiently and maximize your efforts in the shortest amount of time possible.

Each plan is based on the following format: On two alternating days, you'll use lighter weights plus high-intensity training techniques, where your focus is on the lower body for four to five exercises, the upper body for three exercises, and the abs for one exercise. On your second or middle training day, you'll concentrate on using heavier weights and do four to five exercises for the upper body, two lower-body multi-muscle exercises, and two ab exercises. The advanced program includes an optional circuit for the fourth day.

The high-intensity training techniques that you'll be using over the next four weeks are pre-exhaust and the superset or tri-set. These methods will overload your muscles to induce a higher level of tone and definition.

Pre-exhaust

What it is: Pre-exhaust involves performing an isolation move, such as a standing-cable chest fly (which isolates your chest muscles), followed by a multi-muscle move, such as a high-cable chest press (which involves the triceps along with the chest muscles). Or, you can pre-exhaust by doing the multi-muscle exercise first and then finishing with an isolation move. Either way, these can be performed as straight sets or as a superset.

How it works: You begin with an isolation move so that you zero in on a particular muscle group and work it to temporary fatigue. The following multi-muscle exercise targets the same area, along with other muscles to assist it in performing the movement. In contrast, when you begin with the multi-muscle exercise, you'll work the entire group first and then finish with an isolated exercise to finesse the targeted muscle.

Supersets and Tri-Sets

What they are: As mentioned in earlier chapters, a superset means doing two exercises back-to-back without resting until you've completed both exercises. Tri-sets follow the same format with three exercises.

How it works: With either a superset or a tri-set, you focus on the same body part (or related ones) for each exercise. For example, you might do a seated cable high row, which targets your entire upper back and shoulders, followed by a seated bent-over fly, a more isolated exercise which hones in on your deep upper-back muscles.

A superset can also work opposing muscle groups, such as biceps followed by triceps. Muscles are paired, so when one group is working, its partner automatically stretches or lengthens. In this case, if you're doing a biceps exercise, your triceps are stretching, which allows them to be fresh and ready immediately following the first move.

As you perform these high-intensity techniques, you'll find that you probably need to use less weight than if you do straight sets for each individual exercise. That's because you're doing more cumulative work—that is, rather than relying on weight to challenge your muscles, you're using multiple exercises and reps to provide the overload.

Take your time as you practice these techniques, and always be aware of your form. If you're too tired and have difficulty completing the programs, cut back on the number of reps—or even the number of sets—until you improve. You'll discover that the more aware you become of how your body responds and feels, the more control you'll have over your own training success.

The Workouts

As you've seen, the exercises in the body-part chapters you just finished are numbered sequentially: Exercises 1 through 10 are in the abs chapter (page 35), exercises 11 through 20 are in the butt and hips section (page 55), exercises 21 through 30 are in the thighs chapter (page 75), and exercises 31 through 40 are in the upper body chapter (page 97). Keeping this in mind will help you locate precise instructions for the exercises you'll do in this chapter.

These total-body workouts are primarily designed to be done in a gym using machines, although there are some workouts that you can do at home with minimal equipment (such as a set of dumbbells and resistance bands, along with your own body weight). However, if you don't have access to a gym, you can do the at-home options offered in the earlier chapters.

Every workout has a slightly different focus and rotates exercises appropriate for your fitness level, which will help you avoid plateaus and ruts and keep your muscles responding to each and every session. Always warm up with five minutes of light-cardio activity, and complete your workout by stretching the muscles worked, holding each stretch for 30 seconds without bouncing.

You'll progress from beginner to intermediate to advanced after completing each four-week program, or when you're ready to move on to the next level. Repeat the lower-level regimens if your form is poor, you don't feel that you've mastered the moves, or you can't complete the recommended sets or reps with the suggested weight. Even if you're advanced, you might find it beneficial to go back and perform a beginner exercise for variety and to reestablish your form.

We've given you guidelines to follow for each of the three levels, so read them and make sure that you understand the instructions before beginning your workouts.

Beginners

Guidelines: This program includes 3 total-body progressive-strength sessions a week; you'll perform 6–8 exercises each time. By the end of 4 weeks, you should see significant changes in the shape and tone of your body and your overall strength. At that time, you can continue to mix and match these exercises on your own and increase weight or reps, or you can progress to the intermediate program.
Each week, do the exercises in the order listed, resting 45–60 seconds between sets. To complete a superset, do 1 set of each exercise, resting after both exercises, and then repeat the superset.
Rest 45–60 seconds between supersets.

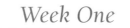

Week One

Do this session on **Days 1 and 3** (say, Monday and Friday).

Exercise	Sets	Reps
21. Wall ball squat	2	8–12
24. Lateral shuffle	1–2	8–12
31. Close grip lat pull-down	2	8–12
36. Seated bent-over rear fly	1–2	8–12
33. Biceps curl	1–2	8–12
11. Forearm side-lying lift and extend	1–2	10–12
1. Basic crunch	2	10–12
5. Obliques rock and reach	1–2	8–12

Do this session on **Day 2** (say, Wednesday).

Exercise	Sets	Reps
22. 3-position leg press	1	6 each position
35. Standing cable chest fly	2	8–12
34. Overhead press	2	8–12
32. High cable press-down	2	8–12

2. High cable crunch	2	8–12
5. Obliques rock and reach	2	8–12

Week Two

Do this session on **Days 1 and 3** (say, Monday and Friday).

Exercise	**Sets**	**Reps**
22. 3-position leg press	1	6–8 each position
35. Standing cable chest fly	2	10–12
32. High cable press-down	2	10–12
13. Sliding plate rear lunge	1–2	6–8
36. Seated bent-over rear fly	2	10–12
24. Lateral shuffle	2	10–12
3. Segmented double crunch	1–2	8–12
4. Stability ball weighted crunch	1–2	8–12

Do this session on **Day 2** (say, Wednesday).

23. Froggies	2	8–12
11. Forearm side lying lift and extend	2	10–15
12. Reverse froggies	2	8–12
31. Close grip lat pull-down	2	10–12
33. Biceps curl	2	10–15
34. Overhead press	2	8–12
1. Basic crunch	2	10–15

Week Three

Do this session on **Days 1 and 3** (say, Monday and Friday). The following moves alternate upper- and lower-body exercises. Perform 1 set of 8–15 reps of each exercise in the order listed without resting in between; this completes 1 circuit. Rest if needed, and repeat the circuit once for a total of 2 circuits.

Exercise	Sets	Reps
21. Wall ball squat	1	8–15
34. Overhead press	1	8–15
13. Sliding plate rear lunge	1	8–15
36. Seated bent-over rear fly	1	8–15
33. Biceps curl	1	8–15
11. Forearm side lift and extend	1	8–15
4. Stability ball crunch	1	8–15

Do this session on **Day 2** (say, Wednesday). Go back to doing the exercises in the order listed, resting 45–60 seconds between sets.

Exercise	Sets	Reps
24. Lateral shuffle	1	10–15
Superset: *22. 3-position leg press*	1–2	8 each position
12. Reverse froggies	1–2	10–15
31. Close grip lat pull-down	2	10–15
35. Standing cable chest fly	2	10–12
32. High cable press-down	2	10–15
2. High cable crunch	2	10–15
3. Segmented double crunch	2	12–15

Week Four

Do this session on **Days 1 and 3** (say, Monday and Friday).
If you're not ready for supersets, just do the exercises in the
order listed, resting 45–60 seconds between sets.

Exercise	**Sets**	**Reps**
Superset: *23. Froggies*	2	8–12
14. One-legged bridge leg extension	2	8–12
Superset: *34. Overhead press*	2	10–12
36. Seated bent-over rear fly	2	8–12
4. Stability ball crunch	2	10–15
Superset: *33. Biceps curl*	2	10–15
32. High cable press-down	2	10–15

Do this session on **Day 2** (say, Wednesday). Go back to doing
the exercises in the order listed, resting 45–60 seconds between sets.

22. 3-position leg press	2	8 each position
31. Close grip lat pull-down	2	8–12
13. Sliding plate lunge	2	8–12
35. Standing cable chest fly	2	10–12
24. Lateral shuffle	2	10–12
1. Basic crunch	2	10–15
5. Obliques rock and reach	2	10–15

Her Ultimate Turning Point

Nicole Frank of South Dakota has a history of weight yo-yoing. Her parents owned a café, and she was a chubby kid as a result of unbridled eating. But by the time she was 15, she'd starved herself down to 103 pounds, which was too thin for her height. Then jobs in a restaurant and a convenience store led to more overeating and weight gain, while a gym membership in college enabled her to use exercise to slim down again. However, that last bout of hard work was undone when she met her future husband and their dates consisted of eating out or making huge home-cooked meals.

At 150 pounds, she decided to commit to getting fit once and for all. She began with healthy eating, and then she took a strength-training course at the gym. "I learned that weight training was an effective way to boost my metabolism and the best way to reach my weight-loss goals," she says. Nicole began working out in this way four days a week, and in two years was 30 pounds lighter. "These days I love what I see in the mirror," she says. "A strong, empowered woman."

Her best tip: Learn basic weight-training techniques through a class, trainer, or fitness magazine (or this book!). It will improve your physique 100 percent.

Intermediate

Guidelines: This program includes 3 total-body progressive-strength sessions a week, plus an optional 4th day of circuit training that you can do at home; you'll perform a maximum of 10 exercises each workout. After 4 weeks or when you're ready, increase from 2 sets to 3—or move on to the advanced program. To complete a superset, do 1 set of each exercise, resting after both exercises, and then repeat the superset. Rest 45–60 seconds between sets and supersets.

Week One

Do this session on **Days 1 and 3** (say, Monday and Friday).

Exercise	Sets	Reps
17. Walking lunges	2–3	10–16
16. Straight-legged bar dead lift	2–3	10–12
18. Step-ups	2–3	10–15
31. Close grip lat pull-down	2–3	8–12
25. Plié/relevé	2–3	10–15
15. Standing ball rear straight leg lift	2–3	10–12
12. Reverse froggies	2–3	10–15
Superset: *33. Biceps curl*	2–3	10–12
38. Bent-over triceps kickback	2–3	10–12
4. Stability ball crunch	2–3	10–15

Do this session on **Day 2** (say, Wednesday).

Exercise	Sets	Reps
22. 3-position leg press	3	8–10 each position
19. Side lunges with dumbbell reaches	2–3	8–12
40. Reciprocal ball chest press	2–3	10–12
32. High cable press-down	2–3	10–15
39. Shoulder fan	2–3	5–6
27. Front-to-back lunge	2–3	10–12
Superset: *37. Seated cable high row*	2–3	8–12
36. Seated bent-over rear fly	2–3	10–12

Exercise	Sets	Reps
7. High to low cable chop	2–3	8–12
3. Segmented double crunch	2–3	10–15

Optional **Day-4** circuit for home or the gym. Do the following moves, alternating upper, middle, and lower body as a circuit. Perform 1 set of 8–15 reps of each exercise in the order listed without resting in between; this completes 1 circuit. Rest if needed, and repeat once for a total of 2 circuits.

Exercise	Sets	Reps
13. Sliding plate rear lunge	1	8–15
34. Overhead press	1	8–15
14. One legged bridge leg extension	1	8–15
8. Arabesque bicycle drops	1	8–15
24. Lateral shuffle	1	8–15
36. Seated bent-over rear fly	1	8–15
28. Skate lunge	1	8–15
9. Forearm plank with knee drops	1	8–15
33. Biceps curl	1	8–15
5. Obliques rock and reach	1	8–15

Week Two

Do this session on **Days 1 and 3** (say, Monday and Friday).

Exercise	Sets	Reps
29. Balanced low cable squat	2–3	10–15
26. Plié jump and drag	2–3	10–12
35. Standing cable chest fly	2–3	10–12
40. Reciprocal ball chest press	2–3	10–12
19. Side lunges with dumbbell reaches	2–3	10–12
24. Lateral shuffle	2–3	8–12
39. Shoulder fan	2–3	5–6
23. Froggies	2–3	10–12

Exercise	Sets	Reps
14. One-legged bridge leg extension	2–3	10–15
6. Weighted bicycle crisscross	2–3	8–12

Do this session on **Day 2** (say, Wednesday).

	Sets	Reps
17. Walking lunges	2–3	10–12
37. Seated cable high row	2–3	10–12
33. Biceps curl	2–3	8–12
32. High cable press-down	2–3	8–12
28. Skate lunge	2–3	10–15
12. Reverse froggies	2–3	10–15
36. Seated bent-over rear fly	2–3	8–12
38. Bent-over triceps kickbacks	2–3	8–12
4. Stability ball crunch	2–3	10–12
7. High-to-low cable chop	2–3	8–12

Optional **Day-4** circuit for home or the gym. Do the following moves, alternating upper, middle, and lower body as a circuit. Perform 1 set of 8–15 reps of each exercise in the order listed without resting in between; this completes 1 circuit. Rest if needed, and repeat once for a total of 2 circuits.

	Sets	Reps
27. Front-to-back lunge	1	8–15
24. Lateral shuffle	1	8–15
34. Overhead press	1	8–15
36. Seated bent-over rear fly	1	8–15
8. Arabesque bicycle drops	1	8–15
25. Plié/relevé	1	8–15
23. Froggies	1	8–15
33. Biceps curl	1	8–15
38. Bent-over triceps kickbacks	1	8–15
9. Forearm plank with knee drops	1	8–15
28. Skate lunge	1	8–15

Week Three

Do this session on **Days 1 and 3** (say, Monday and Friday).

Exercise	Sets	Reps
18. Step-ups	2–3	10–15
27. Front-to-back lunge	2–3	10–15
16. Straight-legged bar dead lift	2–3	10–12
31. Close grip lat pull-down	2–3	8–12
26. Plié jump and drag	2–3	10–16
15. Standing ball rear straight-leg lift	2–3	10–12
Superset: *33. Biceps curl*	2–3	10–12
38. Bent-over triceps kickbacks	2–3	10–12
4. Stability ball crunch	2–3	10–15

Do this session on **Day 2** (say, Wednesday).

Exercise	Sets	Reps
22. 3-position leg press	3	10 each position
19. Side lunges with dumbbell reaches	2–3	10–12
40. Reciprocal ball chest press	2–3	10–12
32. High cable press-down	2–3	12–15
39. Shoulder fan	2–3	5–6
17. Walking lunges	2–3	10–16
Superset: *37. Seated cable high row*	2–3	8–12
36. Seated bent-over rear fly	2–3	8–12
7. High-to-low cable chop	2–3	10–12
3. Segmented double crunch	2–3	10–15

Optional **Day-4** circuit for home or the gym. Do the following moves, alternating upper, middle, and lower body as a circuit. Perform 1 set of 8–15 reps of each exercise in the order listed without resting in between; this completes 1 circuit. Rest if needed, and repeat once for a total of 2 circuits.

Exercise	Sets	Reps
13. Sliding plate rear lunge	1	8–15
34. Overhead press	1	8–15
28. Skate lunge	1	8–15
8. Arabesque bicycle drops	1	8–15
24. Lateral shuffle	1	8–15
36. Seated bent-over rear fly	1	8–15
14. One-legged bridge leg extension	1	8–15
5. Obliques rock and reach	1	8–15
33. Biceps curl	1	8–15
9. Forearm plank with knee drops	1	8–15

Week Four

Do this session on **Days 1 and 3** (say, Monday and Friday).

Exercise	Sets	Reps
29. Balanced low cable squat	2–3	10–15
26. Plié jump and drag	2–3	10–12
35. Standing cable chest fly	2–3	10–12
40. Reciprocal ball chest press	2–3	10–12
19. Side lunges with dumbbell reaches	2–3	10–12
24. Lateral shuffle	2–3	8–12
39. Shoulder fan	2–3	5–6
23. Froggies	2–3	8–12
14. One-legged bridge leg extension	2–3	10–15
6. Weighted bicycle crisscross	2–3	8–12

Do this session on **Day 2** (say, Wednesday).

Exercise	Sets	Reps
17. Walking lunges	2–3	10–12
Superset: 37. *Seated cable high row*	2–3	10–12
33. *Biceps curl*	2–3	10–12
32. High cable press-down	2–3	8–12
28. Skate lunge	2–3	10–15
12. Reverse froggies	2–3	10–15
Superset: 36. *Seated bent-over rear fly*	2–3	8–12
38. *Bent-over triceps kickbacks*	2–3	8–12
4. Stability ball crunch	2–3	10–12
7. High-to-low cable chop	2–3	8–12

Optional **Day-4** circuit for home or the gym. Do the following moves, alternating upper, middle, and lower body as a circuit. Perform 1 set of 8–15 reps of each exercise in the order listed without resting in between; this completes 1 circuit. Rest if needed, and repeat once for a total of 2 circuits.

25. Plié/relevé	1	8–15
24. Lateral shuffle	1	8–15
34. Overhead press	1	8–15
36. Seated bent-over rear fly	1	8–15
9. Forearm plank with knee drops	1	8–15
27. Front-to-back lunge	1	8–15
23. Froggies	1	8–15
38. Bent-over triceps kickbacks	1	8–15
33. Biceps curl	1	8–15
8. Arabesque bicycle drops	1	8–15

Missteps:

- Not being committed. Make sure that you write down your fitness goals, and even tell them to a friend. Once you've declared your intentions, it makes them more real and increases the likelihood that you'll see them through.

- Going it alone. Research shows that you're more likely to stick with your workouts if you have a partner, so pair up with a friend and do the total-body workouts together.

- Getting sloppy. Make sure that you perform each exercise with concentration and control and maintain your alignment, whether you're doing crunches or taking a walk. In other words, 10 perfect reps will take you further toward your Ultimate Body than 50 poorly executed ones.

- Being uncomfortable. Wear workout clothes that are loose, stretchy, or breathable. Avoid all-cotton attire, because its moisture-absorbing properties will make you feel cold and clammy after your workout, regardless of the temperature. Instead, opt for quick-drying poly blends, and always make sure that you have a comfortable sports bra (look for soft, breathable fabrics in polyester/spandex blends with minimal seaming).

- Working too hard. Resting from exercise at least once a week and getting enough sleep (eight to nine hours per night) can increase your fitness benefits and prevent burnout as well.

- Getting bored. Challenge your muscles by trying outdoor activities you may never have considered before, such as rock climbing, kayaking, windsurfing, mountain biking, or cross-country skiing. Discover the playful side of exercise with a game of volleyball, tennis, or golf; or plan an active vacation.

Advanced

Guidelines: This workout includes 3 total-body progressive-strength sessions a week, plus an optional 4th day of circuit training for home or the gym; you'll perform a maximum of 12 exercises each workout. After 4 weeks, you can increase the weight you're lifting in order to up the difficulty level. To complete a superset or tri-set, do 1 set of each exercise, resting after both exercises, and then repeat the superset or tri-set. Rest 45–60 seconds between sets, supersets, and tri-sets.

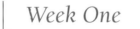

Week One

Do this session on **Days 1 and 3** (say, Monday and Friday).

Exercise		Sets	Reps
Tri-set:	*17. Walking lunges*	2–3	10–16
	16. Straight-legged bar dead lift	2–3	10–12
	18. Step-ups	2–3	10–15
31. Close grip lat pull-down		2–3	8–12
Superset:	*25. Plié/relevé*	2–3	10–15
	15. Standing ball rear straight-leg lift	2–3	10–12
12. Reverse froggies		2–3	10–15

Exercise	Sets	Reps
Superset: *33. Biceps curl*	2–3	10–12
38. Bent-over triceps kickback	2–3	10–12
4. Stability ball crunch	2–3	10–15

Do this session on **Day 2** (say, Wednesday).

Exercise	Sets	Reps
22. 3-position leg press	3	8–10 each position
19. Side lunges with dumbbell reaches	2–3	8–12
Superset: *40. Reciprocal ball chest press*	2–3	10–12
32. High cable press-down	2–3	10–15
39. Shoulder fan	2–3	5–6
27. Front-to-back lunge	2–3	10–12
Superset: *37. Seated cable high row*	2–3	10–12
36. Seated bent-over rear fly	2–3	10–12
7. High-to-low cable chop	2–3	10–12
3. Segmented double crunch	2–3	10–15

Optional **Day 4** circuit for home or the gym. Do the following moves, alternating upper, middle, and lower body as a circuit. Perform 1 set of 10–15 reps of each exercise in the order listed without resting in between; this completes 1 circuit. Rest if needed, and repeat twice for a total of 3 circuits.

Exercise	Sets	Reps
13. Sliding plate rear lunge	1	10–15
34. Overhead press	1	10–15
14. One-legged bridge leg extension	1	10–15
8. Arabesque bicycle drops	1	10–15
24. Lateral shuffle	1	10–15
36. Seated bent-over rear fly	1	10–15
28. Skate lunge	1	10–15
9. Forearm plank with knee drops	1	10–15
33. Biceps curl	1	10–15
5. Obliques rock and reach	1	10–15

Week Two

Do this session on **Days 1 and 3** (say, Monday and Friday).

Exercise		Sets	Reps
Superset:	29. *Balanced low cable squat*	2–3	10–15
	26. *Plié jump and drag*	2–3	10–12
Superset:	35. *Standing cable chest fly*	2–3	10–12
	40. *Reciprocal ball chest press*	2–3	10–12
19. Side lunges with dumbbell reaches		2–3	10–12
24. Lateral shuffle		2–3	8–12
20. Curtsy lunge with side leg lift		2	8–12
39. Shoulder fan		2–3	5–6
23. Froggies		2–3	10–15
14. One-legged bridge leg extension		2–3	10–15
6. Weighted bicycle crisscross		2–3	8–12

Do this session on **Day 2** (say, Wednesday).

Exercise		Sets	Reps
17. Walking lunges		2–3	10–16
Tri-set:	37. *Seated cable high row*	2–3	10–12
	33. *Biceps curl*	2–3	8–12
	32. *High cable press-down*	2–3	8–12
28. Skate lunge		2–3	10–15
30. Kneeling side plank with leg sweeps		2	8–12
12. Reverse froggies		2–3	12–15
36. Seated bent-over rear fly		2–3	10–12
38. Bent-over triceps kickbacks		2–3	8–12
4. Stability ball crunch		2–3	10–15
10. Reverse crunch with knee drops		2–3	8–10

Optional **Day-4** circuit for home or the gym. Do the following moves, alternating upper, middle, and lower body as a circuit. Perform 1 set of 10–15 reps of each exercise in the order listed without resting in between; this completes 1 circuit. Rest if needed, and repeat twice for a total of 3 circuits.

Exercise	Sets	Reps
27. Front-to-back lunge	1	10–15
24. Lateral shuffle	1	10–15
34. Overhead press	1	10–15
36. Seated bent-over rear fly	1	10–15
8. Arabesque bicycle drops	1	10–15
25. Plié/relevé	1	10–15
23. Froggies	1	10–15
33. Biceps curl	1	10–15
38. Bent-over triceps kickbacks	1	10–15
9. Forearm plank with knee drops	1	10–15
28. Skate lunge	1	10–15

Week Three

Do this session on **Days 1 and 3** (say, Monday and Friday).

Exercise		Sets	Reps
Tri-set:	18. Step-ups	2–3	10–15
	27. Front-to-back lunge	2–3	10–15
	16. Straight-legged bar dead lift	2–3	10–12
31. Close grip lat pull-down		2–3	8–12
34. Overhead press		2–3	10–12
Superset:	26. Plié jump and drag	2–3	10–15
	15. Standing ball rear straight leg lift	2–3	10–12
12. Reverse froggies		2–3	12–15
30. Kneeling side plank with leg sweeps		2	8–10

Exercise	Sets	Reps
Superset: *33. Biceps curl*	2–3	10–12
38. Bent-over triceps kickback	2–3	10–12
4. Stability ball crunch	2–3	10–15

Do this session on **Day 2** (say, Wednesday).

Exercise	Sets	Reps
22. 3-position leg press	3	10 each position
19. Side lunges with dumbbell reaches	2–3	10–12
40. Reciprocal ball chest press	2–3	10–12
32. High cable press-down	2–3	12–15
39. Shoulder fan	2–3	5–6
17. Walking lunges	2–3	10–16
29. Balanced low cable squat	2–3	10–12
Superset: *37. Seated cable high row*	2–3	8–12
36. Seated bent-over rear fly	2–3	10–12
7. High-to-low cable chop	2–3	10–15
3. Segmented double crunch	2–3	10–15

Optional **Day-4** circuit for home or the gym. Do the following moves, alternating upper, middle, and lower body as a circuit. Perform 1 set of 10–15 reps of each exercise in the order listed without resting in between; this completes 1 circuit. Rest if needed, and repeat twice for a total of 3 circuits.

Exercise	Sets	Reps
13. Sliding plate rear lunge	1	10–15
34. Overhead press	1	10–15
28. Skate lunge	1	10–15
8. Arabesque bicycle drops	1	10–15
24. Lateral shuffle	1	10–15
36. Seated bent-over rear fly	1	10–15
14. One-legged bridge leg extension	1	10–15
5. Obliques rock and reach	1	10–15
33. Biceps curl	1	10–15
9. Forearm plank with knee drops	1	10–15

Week Four

Do this session on **Days 1 and 3** (say, Monday and Friday).

Exercise		Sets	Reps
Superset:	*29. Balanced low cable squat*	2–3	10–15
	26. Plié jump and drag	2–3	10–12
Superset:	*35. Standing cable chest fly*	2–3	10–12
	40. Reciprocal ball chest press	2–3	10–12
19. Side lunges with dumbbell reaches		2–3	10–12
24. Lateral shuffle		2–3	10–16
20. Curtsy lunge with side leg lift		2	8–12
39. Shoulder fan		2–3	5–6
23. Froggies		2–3	12–15
14. One-legged bridge leg extension		2–3	10–15
6. Weighted bicycle crisscross		2–3	8–12

Do this session on **Day 2** (say, Wednesday).

Exercise		Sets	Reps
17. Walking lunges		2–3	10–15
Superset:	*37. Seated cable high row*	2–3	10–12
	33. Biceps curl	2–3	10–12
32. High cable press-down		2–3	10–12
28. Skate lunge		2–3	10–15
30. Kneeling side plank with leg sweeps		2	8–12
12. Reverse froggies		2–3	10–15
Superset:	*36. Seated bent-over rear fly*	2–3	8–12
	38. Bent-over triceps kickback	2–3	8–12
4. Stability ball crunch		2–3	10–12
10. Reverse crunch with knee drops		2–3	6–8

Optional **Day-4** circuit for home or the gym. Do the following moves, alternating upper, middle, and lower body as a circuit. Perform 1 set of 10–15 reps of each exercise in the order listed without resting in between; this completes 1 circuit. Rest if needed, and repeat twice for a total of 3 circuits.

Exercise	Sets	Reps
25. Plié/relevé	1	10–15
24. Lateral shuffle	1	10–15
34. Overhead press	1	10–15
36. Seated bent over rear fly	1	10–15
9. Forearm plank with knee drops	1	10–15
27. Front-to-back lunge	1	10–15
23. Froggies	1	10–15
38. Bent over triceps kickback	1	10–15
33. Biceps curl	1	10–15
8. Arabesque bicycle drops	1	10–15

Ultimate Word

Add fitness into your daily schedule without feeling like you're working out with these fun sneak-it-in toning tips.

- **Hover squat:** Hover above a chair seat as if you were going to sit down, but without letting your butt or thighs touch the seat. Hold for 30 seconds, building up to 1 minute. Do these whenever you get a moment, aiming for once an hour.

- **Kitchen dip:** Every time you're in the kitchen, perform triceps dips using a kitchen chair. Stand in front of the chair as if you were going to sit down, then bend knees and lower hips, placing hands on the seat edge with fingers pointing forward and arms straight. Walk feet forward, and with feet flat and torso erect, bend and straighten arms, keeping butt close to chair seat without touching it. Do 8–15 reps.

- **Shopping squeeze:** As you push your shopping cart, or whenever you're walking, contract your butt muscles as tightly as you can and keep them contracted as you walk. (No one has to know!)

- **Commercial crunch:** Anytime a commercial comes on while you're watching television, do an ab exercise of your choice until the show you're watching returns; pick a new move for each commercial.

- **Telephone walk:** Whenever you're on a cellular or cordless phone at home, walk around for the duration of the conversation. (Wear a pedometer and see the steps add up.)

- **Balancing act:** When you brush your teeth or while standing at the kitchen sink, lift one leg slightly and bend and straighten your standing leg to perform one-legged squats. Tighten your buttocks and keep your abs contracted as you squat. After 10–15 reps, switch legs and repeat.

In the workouts we've presented so far, we've sometimes called for you to use certain tools or pieces of equipment. Now that you know the moves, we're going to spend the next chapter discussing those exercise aids in greater detail.

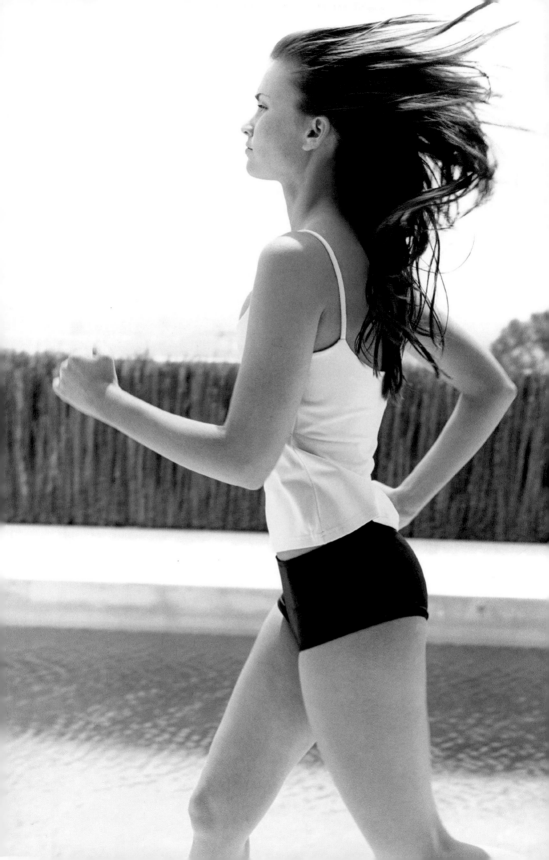

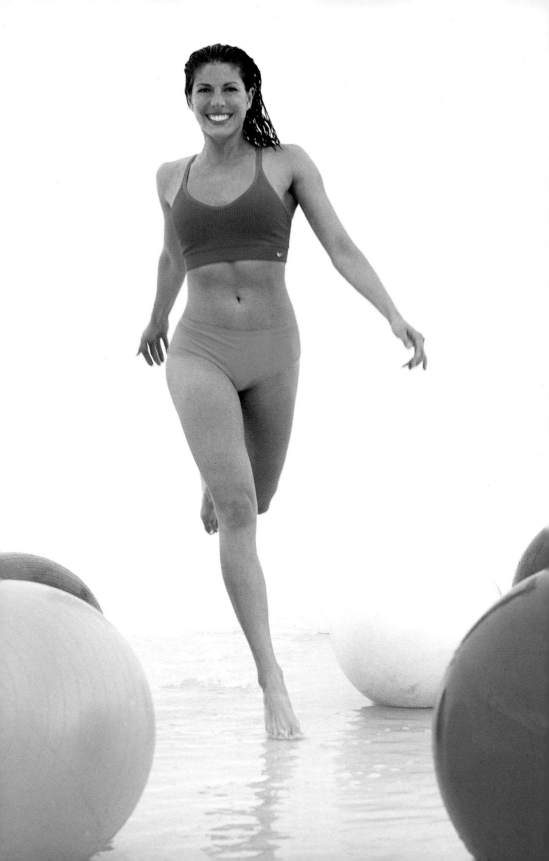

chapter 7

up the ante with tools

Over time, your body will adapt to any exercise routine, so you need to keep working your muscles in new ways in order to see progress. One way to do that is with tools—and what a great variety is available today! Once there were just dumbbells and jump ropes, and perhaps exercise tubing. Now the fitness world has gone ballistic over balls—such as medicine balls and stability balls—and has lost its equilibrium over balance tools. You'll find many of these tools in the gym, or you can use them at home to get better results without adding extra time. (Go to *Shape*'s Website—**www.shape.com**—to find good deals on workout tools.)

This Chapter's To-Do List

In the following pages, you'll learn:

- Why you need tools
- How tone and trim with a medicine ball
- How to sculpt your body by using a stability ball
- The way to boost your muscles and flexibility with balance tools

Are You a "Gearhead"?

You might have read the name of this chapter and thought that you should probably skip it because you really don't need any more tools. Many of you may have unused workout gear sitting in your garage or doubling as a clothes hanger in the bedroom. Maybe you read about some great new piece of equipment or seen some gadget demonstrated on television and splurged—only to regret the impulse later.

If this sounds familiar, ask yourself these questions about the last item you purchased:

1. Did you buy it to keep up with the latest trends or with other people?

2. Do you not understand the instructions, or have you never learned how to use it properly?

3. Did you get it because you were pressured by a salesperson—and now resent it because you couldn't really afford it?

4. Do you feel like you fit in because you have it?

5. Did you think it would make working out easier and require less effort from you?

6. Did you use it for a while, not see immediate results, and then abandon it?

If you answered yes to any of these questions, then you bought the item for the wrong reasons and with unrealistic expectations. The only reason to buy tools is to shake up your routines in order to get more effective results. And you don't need to spend a fortune: The versatile objects in this chapter won't break the bank or take up much space. A relatively small investment can net you increased strength, balance, and coordination; toned muscles; and better posture. And as a bonus, you can have fun while working on your Ultimate Body!

To help you do just that, we'll give you the facts about each of these devices, followed by a series of moves to work different parts of your body. First up is an old standby—and a new favorite.

Medicine-Ball Workout

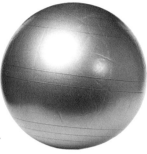

In this program created by renowned trainer Mindy Mylrea of Santa Cruz, California, you'll learn how to use a weighted medicine ball to increase the results of familiar exercises, toning your "show-off zones" without increasing your training time. Medicine balls are old-fashioned exercise tools that have recently rebounded in popularity. They come in various sizes and weights ranging from 2 to 25 pounds in 2- to 5-pound increments, and can cost anywhere from $25 to $100.

Guidelines: Using a 4- to 8-pound medicine ball, do all 8 strength moves in the order shown, 3 days a week on nonconsecutive days. Complete three sets of each exercise, performing the number of reps indicated, before you go on to the next. Rest 45–60 seconds or as needed between sets.

Warm-up: Begin every workout by warming up for 5 minutes with any light-cardio activity.

Cooldown: After each workout, stretch your entire body, holding each stretch to the point of mild tension for 30 seconds without bouncing.

Awesome Abs

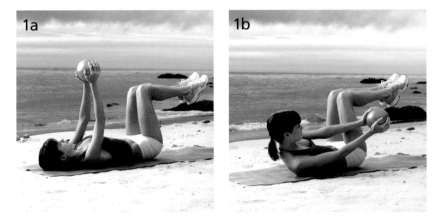

1. Weighted crisscross: Lie on your back with knees bent at 90 degrees and aligned over hips, with calves parallel to the ground. Hold medicine ball above chest, arms extended (a). Contract abs and roll upper back and shoulders off the ground while rotating torso to bring ball toward outside of right knee (b). Keep upper back off the ground as you reach ball over knees and rotate to bring it toward the outside of left knee, keeping hips stable and calves parallel to ground. Lower to starting position and repeat, beginning with the twist first to the left, and then to the right. Continue alternating for 12 reps total.

Strengthens abdominals, with emphasis on obliques.

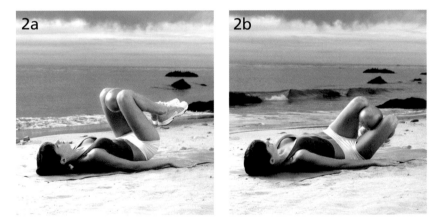

2. Reverse combo crunch: Lie on your back with knees bent, feet on the ground, arms relaxed at sides, and medicine ball between knees. Contract abs, squeeze knees together, and curl butt and hips off the ground, bringing hips toward ribs (a). Roll back down to starting position, your back fully on the ground, then slowly lower knees toward the ground to the right (b). Use abs to bring knees back up to starting position. Repeat, curling hips off the ground and back down, then lowering knees to the left to complete one rep. Do entire move 10 times.

Strengthens abdominals, with emphasis on obliques.

Better Butt and Hips

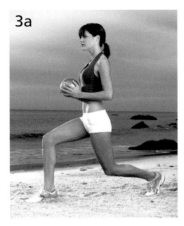

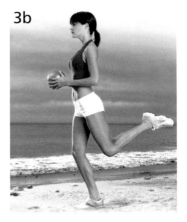

3. Kick-butt lunge: Standing with feet hip-width apart, hold medicine ball in front of chest, with elbows bent at waist. Step forward with right foot into a lunge, bending right knee until it's aligned with right ankle and left knee is pointing toward the ground with heel lifted (a). Plant your weight on right foot and kick left heel back and up toward your buttocks without arching back (b). Then put left foot back down in line with the right, and repeat the entire lunge-kick combo for 12 reps; switch legs and repeat lunges and kicks on opposite side to complete 1 set.

Strengthens buttocks, quadriceps, hamstrings, and calves; inner thighs and upper hips act as stabilizers.

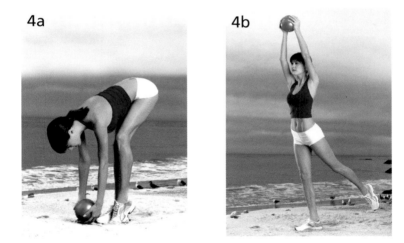

4. Russian lunge, reach, and leg lift: Holding medicine ball in front of chest with elbows bent at waist, stand with left knee slightly bent so that left toes lightly touch the ground. Bend right knee and bend forward from hips while lowering ball toward right foot (a). Straighten right knee and tighten buttocks, bending arms to bring ball back into chest. Then straighten arms overhead as you extend left leg behind you, contracting butt and thigh muscles (b). Lower left toes to ground and ball to chest. Repeat entire move for 10 reps, then switch legs and repeat to complete 1 set.

Strengthens buttocks, quadriceps, hamstrings, upper hips, shoulders, tri-ceps, abdominals, and spine extensors.

Beautiful Upper Body

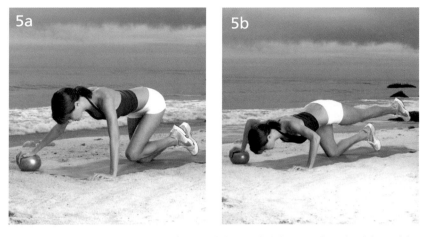

5. Push-up tuck: Kneel on all fours with hands slightly more than shoulder-width apart and slightly forward, left palm flat and right palm on medicine ball. Lift left foot and bend left knee in toward chest (a). Extend left leg behind you; bend elbows and lower torso into a push-up position, aligning elbows with shoulders (b). Straighten arms and repeat tuck and push-up for 5 reps; switch ball to left hand, and tuck with right knee; repeat for 5 reps to complete 1 set.

Strengthens chest, triceps, front shoulders, and buttocks; abdominals and spine extensors act as stabilizers.

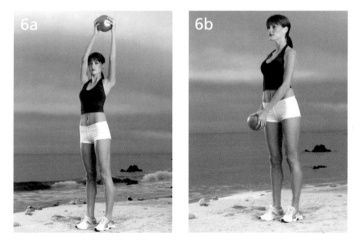

6. X-chop: Standing with feet hip-width apart, knees straight but not locked, hold medicine ball in front of chest, elbows bent at waist. Straighten arms and push the ball to the left and overhead (a). Then, keeping arms straight and without twisting, use middle-back muscles to pull ball down forcefully toward right hip (b). Immediately push ball to the right and overhead, then pull ball down toward left hip. Repeat entire move 12–15 times.

Strengthens front shoulders, chest, rear shoulders, triceps, and middle back.

Tighter Thighs

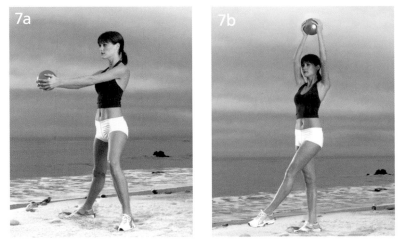

7. Side lunge and sweep: Stand with feet hip-width apart and hold medicine ball with arms straight in front of chest. Step to the left, keeping right leg straight and bending left knee in line with left ankle (a). Push off left foot and sweep left leg across and in front of right leg as you raise ball overhead (b). Return to side lunge and lower arms straight ahead. Repeat entire combo for 10–15 reps, then switch sides and repeat for another 10–15 reps to complete 1 set.

Strengthens inner thighs, upper hips, quadriceps, hamstrings, and buttocks; abdominals act as stabilizers.

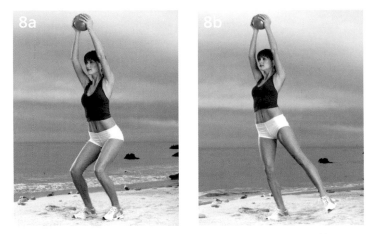

8. Alternating squat kick: Standing with feet hip-width apart and knees straight but not locked, hold medicine ball overhead with arms straight. Tighten abs and then bend knees, aligning them with ankles (a). Straighten knees, then use upper-hip muscles to kick left leg out to left side (b). Pause, then lower left foot to ground and repeat squat, followed by a kick with the opposite leg. Continue alternating legs until you have completed 10 squats total (5 kicks on each side).

Strengthens buttocks, upper hips, quadriceps, and hamstrings; abdominals act as stabilizers.

Q. I see lots of high-tech gadgets out there. Are they worth buying?

A. Gadgets in and of themselves aren't short-cuts to getting fit, but many are very useful for keeping track of your performance, vital signs, and progress. Plus, treating yourself to a fun device can be a useful motivational tool or a reward for meeting a goal. Here are some to try:

- EON Hydra-Alert Watches (from $150; **www.acumeninc.com**) gauge your exertion, along with the temp-erature and humidity, enabling you to accurate-ly assess your hydration needs as you exercise.

- Caltrac ($70; **www.caltrac.net**) looks like a clip-on pager but actually informs you of the number of calories you're torching wherever you go. Enter the amount of calories you've eaten throughout the day to see if you've burned more than you've consumed.

- Duel Sports Digital Music Player/ Heart Rate Monitor ($280; **www. digisette.com**) is a combination heart-rate monitor, FM radio, and shock- and skip-proof MP3 audio player that's easy to use.

- Forerunner 201 GPS system ($160; **www.garmin.com**) is a small, light-weight device that fits onto your wrist like a watch but can calculate speed, distance, pace, and calorie burn. In addition, it provides precise latitude, longitude, and altitude data to help you determine your exact location.

Stability-Ball Workout

Stability balls (also called "physioballs" or "Swiss balls") are large balls originally designed for physical therapy. Working out with this tool is an incredible way to sculpt your entire body. It also challenges your balance, which is ideal for strengthening your core muscles—the abs in particular.

"Strengthening your core assists in injury prevention and helps your body function more efficiently," adds Beverly Hills–based trainer-to-the-stars Gunnar Peterson.

Guidelines: Do this circuit-style program 2–3 times a week, taking a day off between workouts. Perform 1 set of Moves 1–4 in the order listed without resting between exercises, and then repeat before transitioning to Moves 5–8, which you'll repeat as well. Use enough weight to fatigue your target muscles by the final rep of each set, where applicable. To increase the intensity, switch to heavier dumbbells or aim for the higher number of reps recommended. If you're a beginner or have trouble with balance, do the workout without dumbbells until you feel comfortable with it. You may also want to use a ball that isn't fully inflated (which will be less challenging).

Equipment: For this workout, you'll need 2 pairs (1 lighter pair and 1 heavier pair) of 5- to 10-pound dumbbells and a stability ball. Most women over 5'4" will need a 65-centimeter ball; if you're under this height, try a 55-centimeter one. Your knees should be bent at a 90-degree angle when you're seated on top of the ball.

Warm-up: Begin each workout by sitting on the ball and gently bouncing for one minute. Then face the ball, bend knees into a squat, pick up ball, and straighten legs as you lift it overhead; bend knees into another squat as you lower arms to return ball to ground. Repeat 10 times.

Cooldown: End each workout by stretching all of your major muscle groups, holding each stretch for 20–30 seconds without bouncing.

Cardio: Do 25–45 minutes of aerobic activity 3–5 days a week. For best results, vary the activities, time, and intensity.

The Moves

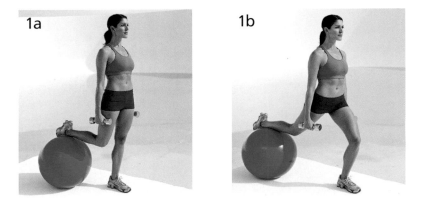

1. Ball lunge: Stand with ball a few inches behind you, dumbbells hanging at your sides in each hand, palms facing in. Then place top of right foot on top of ball, right knee bent, abs contracted and chest lifted (a). If necessary, hold a chair or wall for support. Adjust left foot as far forward as necessary to be in a split stance (one long stride in front of right foot). Keeping torso centered between legs and left knee aligned with left ankle, bend left knee into a lunge, pressing down slightly on ball with right foot as you extend right leg as far back as possible while lowering right knee toward ground (b). Straighten left leg, pulling ball toward you with right leg, and repeat for 10–16 reps. Switch legs and repeat.

Strengthens quadriceps, hamstrings, and buttocks; abdominals, spine extensors, inner thighs, and upper hips work as stabilizers.

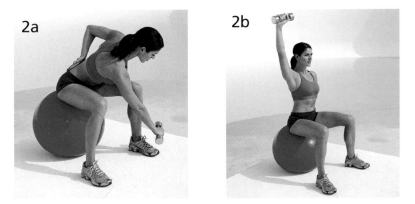

2. Cross row: Holding a dumbbell in your right hand, sit on ball with knees bent and feet flat on the ground, ankles in line with knees, left hand on the small of back. Keeping abs contracted and hips square, bend forward from hips and extend right arm so that dumbbell is near the outside of left foot, palm facing in (a). Bend elbow back and up in a rowing motion as you sit back up to an erect position and straighten arm overhead (b). Lower arm and repeat entire movement for 6–8 reps. Switch sides and repeat.

Strengthens middle and upper back, shoulder, abdominals, and spine extensors.

3a

3b

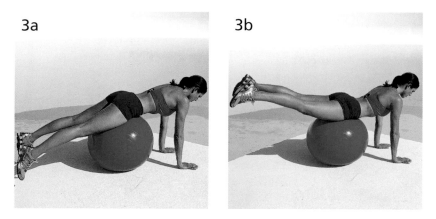

3. Reverse hyper: Kneel with torso draped over ball, facedown, then walk hands forward until you're in a plank position with front of hips and thighs on top of ball, wrists in line with shoulders. Separate feet and rotate hips outward so feet hover a few inches above ground (a). Keeping hands planted on floor, contract buttocks to lift legs up to hip height (b). Lower to starting position and repeat for 12–16 reps.

Strengthens buttocks and hamstrings; abdominal and spine extensors work as stabilizers.

4a

4b

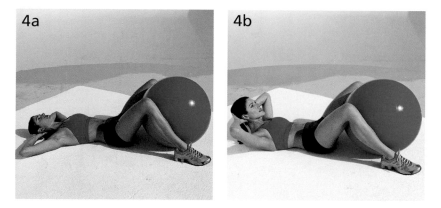

4. Ab crunch: Lie faceup, grasping ball between bent knees, feet flat on the floor. Place unclasped fingertips behind head or hold 1 dumbbell in both hands on chest. Contract abs to bring spine into a neutral position (a). Squeeze ball with inner thighs while lifting head, neck, and shoulder blades up off floor (b). Slowly lower and repeat for 12–16 reps.

Strengthens abdominals and inner thighs.

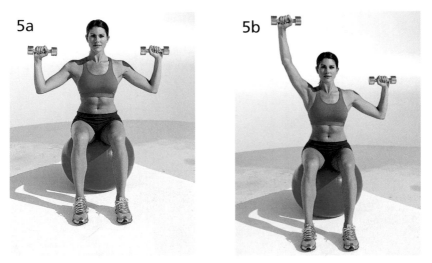

5. Alternate shoulder press: Holding a dumbbell in each hand, sit on ball with knees bent, ankles in line with knees. Hold each dumbbell just above shoulder height, elbows bent, palms facing forward, abs contracted, chest lifted, and shoulders relaxed (a). Staying erect, press right arm straight overhead without locking elbow (b). Lower dumbbell back to just above shoulder height, then repeat on left side. Continue alternating sides to complete 6–8 reps on each side.

Strengthens middle and front shoulders, upper and middle back, and abdominals.

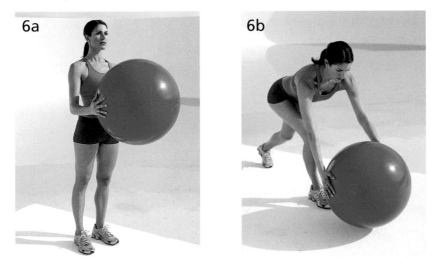

6. Elvis lunge: Stand holding ball in front of torso with elbows bent and feet hip-width apart. Contract abs, drawing tailbone down so that spine is in a neutral position (a). Step forward with right foot, bending both knees so that right knee is aligned over right ankle and left heel is lifted as you bend forward as if to put ball down on the floor in front of you, keeping back straight (b). Push back to starting position, picking up ball. Alternate lunges to complete 6–8 reps on each side.

Strengthens quadriceps, hamstrings, buttocks, calves, abdominals, spine extensors, middle and upper back, shoulders, and arms.

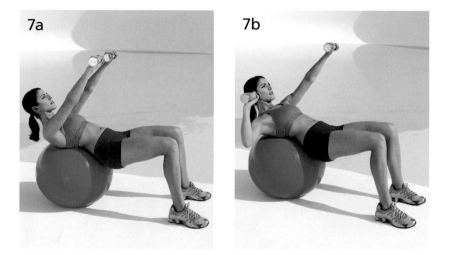

7. Incline one-arm chest press: Holding a dumbbell in each hand, lie faceup with middle and lower back supported on ball, knees bent, feet flat on the floor, and hips lower than chest. Extend arms above chest, palms facing forward (a). Bend right elbow, lowering arm until elbow aligns with right shoulder, wrist in line with dumbbell; keep left arm lifted (b). Straighten right arm back to starting position and repeat for 6–8 reps before switching sides.

Strengthens chest, front shoulders, and triceps.

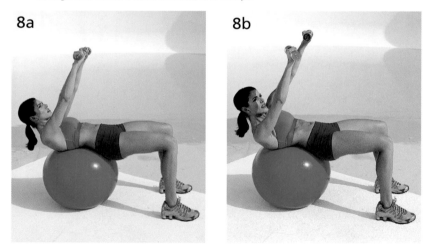

8. Crunch with punch: Lie faceup with middle and lower back supported on ball, knees bent. Hold a dumbbell in each hand with arms extended above chest and abs contracted so that spine is in a neutral position (a). Inhale, then exhale while lifting head and shoulders into a crunch position, simultaneously pushing left dumbbell as far up as possible, palms down (b). Slowly alternate "punches" to complete 6–10 reps on each side.

Strengthens abdominals, chest, and front shoulders.

Her Ultimate Turning Point

By the time she turned 29, Donna Cutignola of New Jersey weighed 230 pounds and had accepted that she'd be heavy for life. But her sister, who wanted to lose weight, challenged Donna to do it, too. Although they lived in different states, they agreed to call each other once a week to check on each other's progress. By following a healthy diet, Donna lost 50 pounds (her sister lost 15 before becoming pregnant and putting her program on hold). At 180 pounds, Donna decided to start exercising, but "I felt too big to work out at a gym and instead bought an aerobics video," she says. It took her seven tries over a two-week period to get through the entire 60-minute routine. But exercise was what she needed, and the weight started coming off at a rate of five pounds a month. Next she invested in a step-aerobics tape and dumbbells. "As my weight loss continued," she says, "my family and friends were astonished by the changes in me—physically and mentally. I felt like I was 20 again." She reached her goal weight of 120 pounds a year and a month after starting.

Her Best Tip: Make exercise a part of your routine. Schedule time to do it and stick with it.

Balance-Tools Moves

If you'd like to get more impressive results from your workouts without adding extra time, we've got a simple and speedy solution: Start using balance tools, like a wedge, foam block, or air-filled disc. By combining dumbbell moves with cushy equipment, you increase the workout challenge and the payoff.

You see, when you step onto an unstable surface, your body has to work to stay balanced—so you naturally use more muscles than just the ones you're targeting. Strengthening these stabilizer muscles (such as the quadriceps, hamstrings, upper hips, inner thighs, and core muscles) reduces your risk of injury and helps you perform everyday activities with greater ease. Plus, you'll look slimmer and more sculpted from head to toe.

In addition to dumbbells, you'll need a piece of balance equipment to perform this program designed by Charleene O'Connor, a certified personal trainer and fitness director at Clay, a fitness club in New York City. In our pictures, we've used three different ones: the foam BodyWedge21 that costs around $20; a nubby air-filled Xerdisc, about $35; and a soft Airex Balance Pad, around $40. If you want to invest in only one, the BodyWedge21 is perhaps the most versatile, because you can use the lower end when a disc or balance pad is recommended.

You may choose to buy nothing at all. To start, you can perform most of these moves on an unstable surface such as a couch cushion placed on the floor. Just do this workout consistently as prescribed and you'll get a sleeker, stronger physique in less time than you'd expect.

Guidelines: Do this workout twice a week with 1 or 2 days off in between. Begin with 2 sets of 10–15 reps of each move in the order listed, resting 60 seconds between sets. When you're ready, you can progress to 3 sets or increase the weight enough to challenge your muscles without disrupting your balance. For safety, do this workout on a nonslippery surface or place a sticky yoga mat under the equipment.

Beginners Rx: If you haven't strength trained in 3 months or more, or you've never used balance tools or done these particular dumbbell exercises before, simply perform this workout standing on the floor *without* the balance tools. Once you've learned proper form and alignment and feel that you can keep your balance on an unstable surface, progress to doing 1 set of exercises on the floor and 1 set on the balance tools *without* dumbbells. After 3 or 4 weeks, you should be able to do the entire workout using all equipment as prescribed.

Warm-up: Begin by marching or jogging in place for 5 minutes, or jump rope for 5 minutes using a boxer's shuffle. Then do side-to-side hops—one foot at a time—to warm up your ankles. Finally, stand erect on one of the balance tools and lift one foot slightly, rotating it 20 times in each direction; then do the same with the other foot.

Cooldown: Complete your workout by stretching your major muscles, holding each stretch for 30 seconds without bouncing.

Cardio: Aim to do 30–45 minutes of aerobic exercise 3 to 5 days per week, doing a mix of steady-state and interval training to challenge your cardiovascular system and burn more calories.

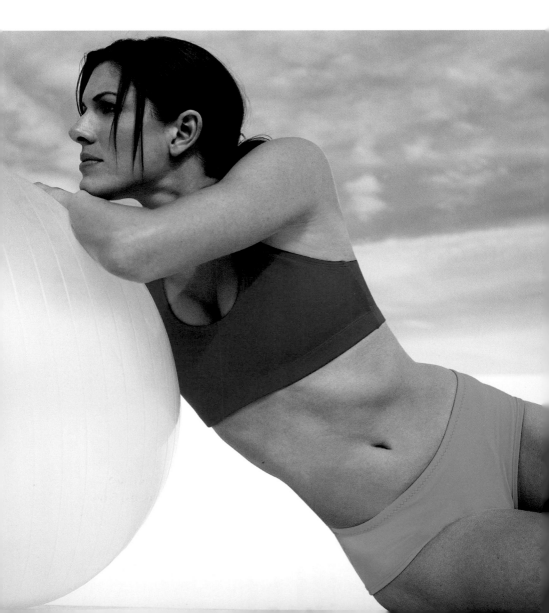

Misstep:

Not taking safety precautions when using balance tools.
For safety and improved results, avoid these mistakes
when using any piece of balance equipment.
Don't . . .

- Move too quickly; this is an easy way to lose your
  balance.

- Perform jumping or other exercises that require explosive
  movement on balance tools unless you're extra cautious;
  this requires even more stability and control and may
  lead to injury if you're not experienced with working out
  on unstable surfaces.

- Cheat by frequently putting your hands or feet down
  to reestablish your balance (unless you're in danger of
  falling); this minimizes the effectiveness of the exercise.

- Put balance tools on an unstable surface like a slippery
  floor; this can lead to injury.

- Forget to keep contracting your abdominal muscles as
  you perform each rep; not contracting them is a primary
  reason you lose your balance.

- Use as much weight as you would when doing resistance
  exercises on a stable surface; this can compromise your
  form.

The Moves

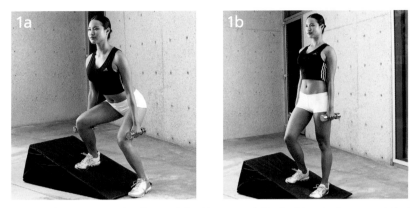

1. Side squat: Stand with your right side to a BodyWedge21 at the lowest end, feet slightly apart, and hands on hips or holding a dumbbell in each hand with arms hanging at sides. Contract abs and step sideways with right foot so that feet are hip-width apart, right foot on wedge, and bending knees to squat while keeping body weight toward heels (a). Straighten legs and bring left foot onto wedge toward right foot (b). Continue to sidestep and squat until you've gone all the way up to the top of the wedge; then sidestep and squat down, leading with left foot. At the bottom, turn around and repeat, leading up the wedge with left leg and down with right leg to complete 1 set.

Weight: 5- to 10-pound dumbbells.

Strengthens quadriceps, hamstrings, buttocks, upper hips, and inner thighs.

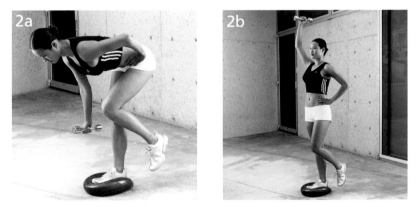

2. Single straight-leg dead lift, curl, and press: Stand on an Xerdisc with right foot, right leg straight, and left leg bent with foot slightly lifted. Hold a dumbbell in right hand, arm hanging at side, palm in, and left hand on left hip. Keeping right leg straight, bend forward at hips with back straight, until torso is parallel to floor and right arm is hanging down near lower leg, close to body (a). Return torso to stand erect and bend right elbow to bring dumbbell up to right shoulder in a hammer curl (palm still in), then press arm straight overhead (b). Bend elbow to bring dumbbell to shoulder, then lower dumbbell to side and immediately repeat dead lift, curl, and press. Do reps, then switch sides to complete 1 set.

Weight: 5- to 8-pound dumbbell.

Strengthens hamstrings, buttocks, spine extensors, biceps, front and middle shoulders, and upper back.

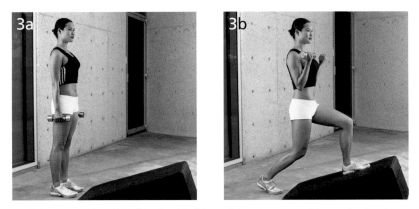

3. Lunge and curl: Hold a dumbbell in each hand, arms at sides, and palms in. Stand facing a BodyWedge21 at the lowest end, feet hip-width apart, abs contracted and torso erect (a). Take a large step forward onto the wedge with one foot, bending both knees so that front knee aligns with front ankle and back knee approaches floor, back heel lifted. As you lunge, bend both elbows, rotating palms up while bringing dumbbells to shoulders (b). Step back to starting position, straightening arms down and rotating palms in. Repeat with opposite leg to complete 1 rep. Continue alternating legs to complete the set.

Weight: 5- to 10-pound dumbbells.

Strengthens quadriceps, hamstrings, buttocks, calves, and biceps.

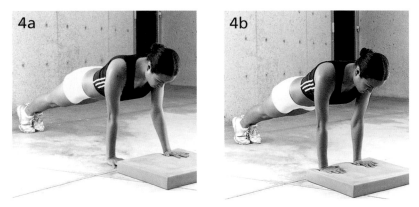

4. Plank walk-up: Kneel on all fours with hands flat on the floor just behind an Airex Balance Pad, wrists under shoulders and knees under hips. Extend legs one at a time behind you, balancing on balls of feet with legs together. Contract abs so that body forms one straight line from head to heels. Maintain plank while lifting left hand and placing it flat onto the pad, keeping shoulders over wrists (a), then right hand (b). Lift and return right hand to starting position, then left hand to complete 1 rep. Continue walking hands up-up, down-down, keeping abs tight and body straight in plank position. Repeat, changing lead arm every 5 reps until you complete the set.

Strengthens abdominals, spine extensors, chest, shoulders, triceps; buttocks and all leg muscles work as stabilizers.

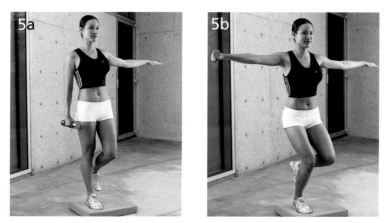

5. Single-leg squat with lateral raise: Stand in the center of an Airex Balance Pad with right leg straight, left foot slightly lifted and close to right calf. Hold a dumbbell in right hand, arm hanging at side, elbow in a slight arc, palm in, and abs contracted. Extend left arm out to the side at shoulder height, palm down, for balance (a). Bend right knee, sitting back into a squat, while at the same time lifting right arm up and out to shoulder height (b). Straighten right leg and lower right arm. Repeat squat and raise for recommended number of reps, then switch legs and working arm and repeat to complete the set.

Weight: 3- to 5-pound dumbbell.

Strengthens buttocks, hamstrings, quadriceps, middle shoulder; upper hip and inner thigh of squatting leg work as stabilizers.

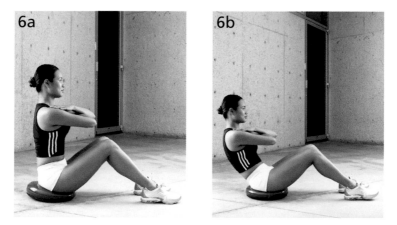

6. Ab balance: Sit erect on an Xerdisc, knees bent and feet flat on the floor. Keep legs squeezed together and arms crossed over chest (a)—or, for a greater challenge, place fingertips behind head. Contract abs and tilt pelvis to curl torso back and down toward floor; only go as low as you can while keeping feet firmly on the floor (b). Keep spine rounded as you curl back up to a sitting position, and repeat.

Strengthens abdominals and spine extensor.

Your Toolbox

Apart from those tools specifically mentioned in the workouts in this chapter, there are a number of other products that you can add to your Ultimate Body toolbox.

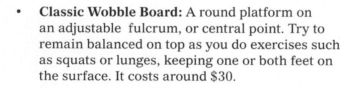

- **BOSU Balance Trainer:** This is half of a stability ball attached to a level base. You can stand, sit, or lean on the dome side; or flip it over for an even more intense challenge. It costs around $100, which includes a pump, an exercise manual, and a how-to video.

- **Reebok Core Board:** A plastic platform on an adjustable base that tilts, rocks, and swivels. Balance on top as you perform strength moves such as biceps curls and overhead presses. It costs around $150.

- **Classic Wobble Board:** A round platform on an adjustable fulcrum, or central point. Try to remain balanced on top as you do exercises such as squats or lunges, keeping one or both feet on the surface. It costs around $30.

- **Xertube Resistance Bands:** Tubes with handles that are great for home or on-the-road workouts. They're color coded (yellow, green, red, blue, and purple) in ascending levels of intensity—so beginners would choose yellow, while elite athletes would pick purple. Get three different tubes for around $15, or a kit with an instructional video for $30.

- **Body Bar:** A 2- to 6-foot-long weighted bar with padding; comes in weights ranging from 4 to 36 pounds. Use like a barbell to do moves such as squats, upright rows, and biceps curls. It costs $23 to $90, depending on weight.

Ultimate Word

Can sitting on a stability ball rather than on a chair in the office help firm abs? According to Elizabeth Larkam, M.A., at Western Athletic Clubs in San Francisco, it's unlikely. "When you sit on an unstable surface, your abs and the muscles around your spine have to work harder just to keep you steady," she explains. "But you won't get the intensity of muscle contraction that you need to see a difference in abdominal tone." For that you need to do your ab moves. Sitting on a ball *can* help improve your posture, although you still need to pay attention to how you're sitting. "It's possible to slump on a ball, just as it's possible to slump in a chair," says Larkam. "Make sure that you aim your 'sit bones'—the bones at the bottom of your pelvis that you sit on—directly down to the floor. And as you balance your hips on the ball, think about balancing your rib cage directly above them."

Larkam recommends sitting on a ball for 5–10 minutes at a time. Be aware that you need to choose the right size ball for your height: If you're over 5'4" tall, you'll probably need a 65-centimeter ball, as opposed to one that measures 55 centimeters. When seated, your knees should form a 90-degree angle.

All of these workouts with different tools can really help you achieve your Ultimate Body in short order. But if you'd like to see changes and get back to the basics of feeling your body, you'll enjoy the next chapter, where we'll give you the best yoga and Pilates moves to tighten and tone your muscles

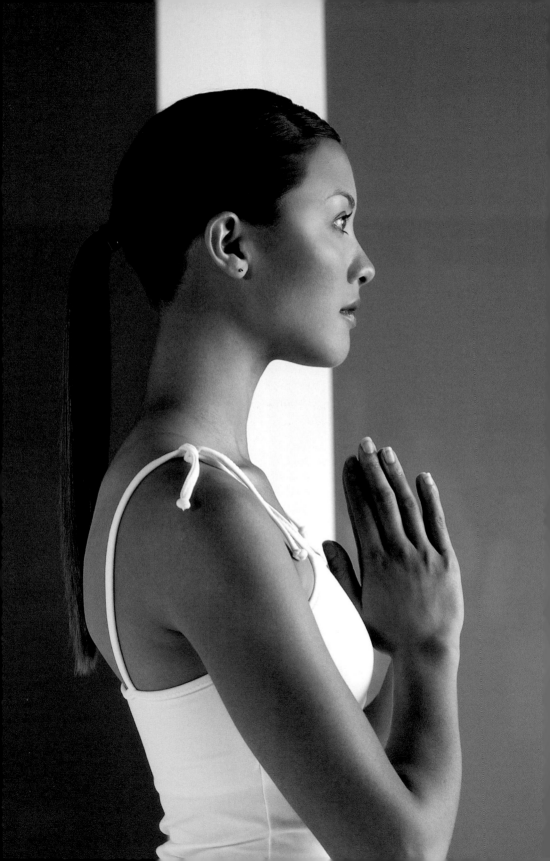

chapter 8

yoga and pilates

Yoga has been around as a spiritual practice for 5,000 years, yet its recent popularity might have seemed to be a fleeting fitness trend for the "stretchy-feely" set. Instead, yoga is proving to have staying power in the Western world, not just for its ability to calm the mind, but also for the way it strengthens the body. Pilates, on the other hand, dates back less than 100 years, but it's meeting with as much success as the older discipline—perhaps because both have so much to offer in our frenetic, fast-paced, 21st-century lifestyles.

This Chapter's To-Do List

In these pages, you'll learn:

- What yoga and Pilates have in common
- How yoga can calm or energize you, depending on your needs
- Ways to get flat abs with these moves
- Intense calorie-burning regimens
- Tips for getting the maximum results from your workouts

Two of a Kind

Yoga and Pilates are paired together here, much as they are in many gym classes, because they have much in common. Both of these disciplines do the following:

- Train from the "inside out." They require that you generate all movement from your center (or core) with precision.

- Enhance everyday movement. When doing these exercises, you use abdominal and back muscles to support and stabilize your body as you work through many planes and angles of movement, just as you do in life. This improves your ability to perform virtually any activity, enhances suppleness, and optimizes muscle and joint functioning, which is also anti-aging.

- Improve balance. When your ab and back muscles work together, the mobility and extension of your spine are increased so that you move more fluidly and gracefully.

- Promote quality over quantity. Yoga and Pilates encourage you to concentrate on how purposefully and precisely you can perform each pose, rather than on how many reps you can do, so you're less likely to use momentum and speed to execute an exercise. You actually learn to move your muscles the way that they're intended to, which may help prevent injury.

Two-in-One Yoga Stress-Buster

Stress is almost inevitable these days. Too many commitments to family and friends, lack of sleep, work demands, and other obligations may leave you too exhausted to exercise or so anxious and agitated that the last thing you want to do is head to a crowded gym.

Whether you need an energy boost or that peaceful, easy feeling, this two-in-one at-home yoga workout can help. "Depending on how you practice the routine, you can actually change the quality of your energy, and go from being tense to tranquil, or drained to revitalized," explains Rome, Georgia–based Leigh Crews, the National Academy of Sports Medicine–certified trainer and yoga instructor who created this program.

But first take our "Stress-Detector Test" to find out which workout—the energy-boosting or the energy-calming program, or both—will benefit you most. Then follow the prescribed regimen for improved energy levels and a more beautiful body.

Stress-Detector Test

Everyone reacts differently to the stressors in life, which can take a toll on your mind and body. Perhaps you feel too agitated to exercise, maybe you get so tired that you turn to sugary snacks to perk yourself up, or it could be that you repress these feelings or experience a combination of the two. Take this quiz to find out whether you need to calm down or get fired up—or both!

1. Stress makes you feel:
   a. Overly sensitive, panicked, scattered, crabby, short-tempered, and impatient.
   b. Exhausted, apathetic, drained, emotionless, passionless, and desperate for a nap.
   c. Too tired to concentrate, but too tense to sleep or truly relax.

2. Stress makes you physically:
    a. Agitated, jittery, ill at ease.
    b. Incapacitated—any kind of activity,
        including taking a walk, seems impossible.
    c. Tense—you feel pain in your head, neck,
        shoulders, or spine, and are short of breath.
        You may even feel your heart palpitating
        or muscles twitching.

If you answered "a" to both questions, you're a high-strung stress reactor. You have excess energy to burn, so you need a vigorous workout of at least 20 minutes that will release tension and help sharpen your focus. Begin with the Full-Sun Breaths warm-up, then follow instructions for the Energy-Boosting routine, which alternates flowing and held postures. This will pump up your heart rate, increase your stamina, and power your aerobic system so that you can release pent-up tension and stress and feel more balanced. Finish with the Energy-Calming routine to release any remaining agitation, and end with the cooldown as instructed.

If you answered "b" to both questions, you're a run-down stress reactor. When faced with too much pressure, you feel exhausted and don't have an ounce of energy left, so you need to get revitalized at a slower, more progressive pace. Rather than warming up with the Full-Sun Breaths, begin with the Energy-Calming routine and then do the Full-Sun Breaths to gradually increase your energy.

Next, assess whether you've perked up enough to move on to the Energy-Boosting routine—or if you feel sufficiently energized, you can stop there and simply end with the cooldown as instructed.

If you answered "c" to both questions—or a combination of all three choices—you're a stressor repressor: When you feel overwhelmed, you shut down and internalize your tension, so you need a relaxing routine to help relieve stress. Begin with the Full-Sun Breaths warm-up. The repetitive activity, along with regular inhalations and exhalations, will give you the even-keeled energy that you need. Then do the Energy-Calming routine, which will continue to instill a feeling of serenity and grounding. End with the cooldown, staying in corpse pose and breathing for as long as it takes for your muscles to relax and your brain to quiet down.

Guidelines: Use either the Energy-Boosting routine or the Energy-Calming routine as often during the week as you like to invigorate and/or soothe yourself.

Warm-up: Begin either routine with Full-Sun Breaths, unless you're a run-down stress reactor.

Cooldown: After you've completed 1 or both routines, relax in corpse pose: Lie on your back, letting feet fall open with arms relaxed at sides, palms up. Breathe deeply, inhaling and exhaling down into your belly, expanding and closing your rib cage with each breath. Stay here as long as you like.

If you choose to do only the Energy-Boosting routine, complete 2 cycles of Full-Sun Breaths very slowly to bring your heart rate down; then stand with eyes closed in mountain pose for 4–6 breaths.

Cardio and strength training: While this workout will get your heart rate up, rev your energy, sculpt your muscles, and bust stress, it shouldn't be used as a substitute for a regular aerobic or strength-training program. Aim to complete 3–5 days of cardio and 1–2 total-body strength workouts a week as well.

Q. **My yoga mat is getting pretty funky. How can I clean it?**

A. Some yoga mats come with instructions for machine washing (minus the spin cycle), but according to San Diego–based Mara Carrico, yoga spokesperson for the American Council on Exercise, you're better off keeping it out of the washer. "Total submersion may get your mat clean," Carrico says, "but it can take up to a month to fully dry. And never put your mat in the dryer."

Carrico suggests using a mild antibacterial soap or a mixture of ⅓ water, ⅓ white vinegar, and ⅓ rubbing alcohol in a spray bottle. "Spray your mat and rub it down with a sponge, terry cloth, or plastic scrubber," she instructs. "Then roll it between two towels to dry, and air it out someplace that has good air circulation but is out of the direct sun." Carrico adds that simply unrolling your yoga mat and "letting it breathe" every so often will also help.

In addition, there are some commercial products that you can spray on your mat after using it that claim to have antibacterial and deodorizing effects.

Full Sun Breaths

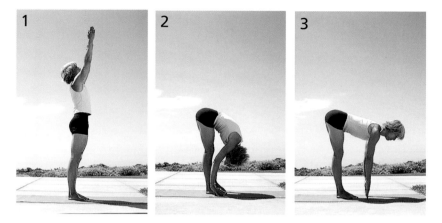

Start in mountain pose. Inhale, sweeping arms up overhead and keeping arms slightly apart and parallel (1). Exhale, "hinge" over at hips into a forward bend, stretching arms and head toward the floor while keeping legs straight or slightly bent; let spine round (2). Inhale and look forward, placing fingertips on the ground or on shins, elongating spine so that it's straight (3).

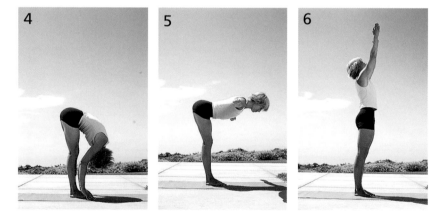

Exhale and return to forward bend, rounding spine (4). Inhale, bending knees if necessary, sweeping arms out to sides (5), then up and overhead as you move back up to mountain pose and straighten legs (6). Exhale and return arms to sides.

The Energy-Boosting Routine

Do the following moves in the order listed, alternating between flowing or "vinyasa-style" poses (1, 3, and 5) and holding poses (2 and 4). For moves 1, 3, and 5, flow between the "a" and "b" parts without stopping, exhaling for 4–6 counts to get into each position and inhaling for 4–6 counts to get out of it. Repeat each of these moves 4–8 times. For poses 2 and 4, hold each for 3–5 complete breaths in order to increase your stamina and strength and refocus your mind. Return to mountain pose between all moves.

Mountain pose: You'll begin each of the moves for this routine in this position. Stand with big toes together, heels slightly apart, and legs straight. Place thumbs against breastbone with palms together and elbows bent. Draw shoulder blades down, tighten thigh muscles, pull belly in, and keep tailbone pointing toward the floor.

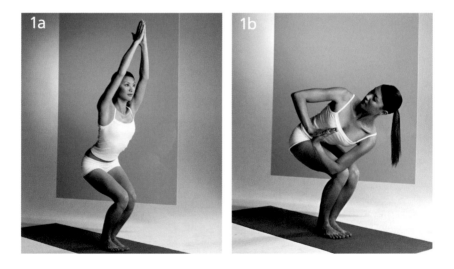

1. Rotating chair: From mountain pose, inhale while extending arms overhead. Keeping palms, knees, ankles, and feet together, bend both knees as if sitting in a chair (a). Then bring left elbow to outside of right thigh, exhaling as you rotate torso and look back at right elbow (b). Inhale while straightening legs and extending arms overhead to return to starting position. Repeat on opposite side.

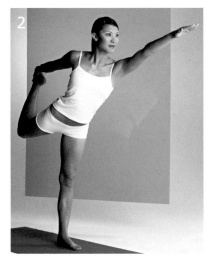

2. Dancer: From mountain pose, extend left arm up with palm down. Bend right knee, bringing right foot up behind butt, and grasp the top of foot or ankle with right hand. Draw tailbone down so that spine is in a neutral position, and tighten thighs. Bend slightly forward from hips, reaching left arm and right foot away from each other, creating strong tension between right leg and upper body, as shown. Hold for recommended breaths, then stand back up, releasing right foot to floor, and repeat on opposite side.

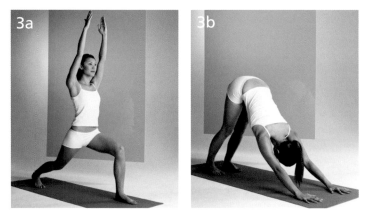

3. Lunge vinyasa: From mountain pose, inhale; then exhale and step forward with left foot, bending knees so that left foot aligns with left ankle, keeping right knee slightly bent and heel lifted. Inhale while extending arms overhead (a). Exhale and bend forward from hips, placing one hand on each side of left foot. Step left foot back to meet right, straightening legs and lifting hips up in an inverted V. Press thighs back and chest down so that heels are as close to floor as possible (downward-facing-dog pose) (b).

Inhale and look through your hands; then exhale and step forward with your right foot this time, inhaling as you stand erect and lift arms overhead to repeat lunge on opposite side.

Misstep:

Not inhaling and exhaling correctly. Use of the breath is a key element of both yoga and Pilates, helping you stabilize your spine, move deeper into a pose, or calmly maintain the one you're already in. While there's a slight difference between the breathing technique used in yoga and the one used in Pilates, the goal is the same: to get the most from your breath. Keep these pointers in mind:

- Don't hold it. As you work your abs to maintain alignment in each pose, focus on keeping your breathing calm and even.

- Work with it. Use your breath to help you stay firm in your middle by keeping consistent tension in your abs.

- Go deep. Initiate the breath from deep in your diaphragm, not from your chest.

- Open and close. When you inhale, visualize your rib cage expanding; when you exhale, think of a purposeful release while contracting your abs.

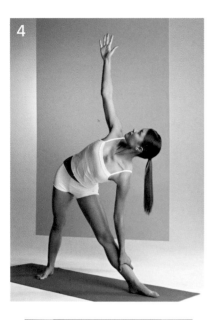

4. Triangle: From mountain pose, step back about 3–4 feet with right foot, turning right toes out 30 degrees and aligning left heel with right arch. Open hips to the right so that body is square, and lift arms to shoulder height, palms down. Exhale, keeping legs straight, and shift torso over left leg, tilting left hip down so that torso is sideways and nearly parallel to the floor. Continue to rotate right hip out (to keep hips open) and raise right hand overhead, placing left hand on left shin. Look up at right hand, as shown. Stay in this position for the recommended number of breaths. Then inhale, lifting torso back to an upright position. Turn feet and torso the other way, and repeat on opposite side.

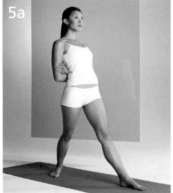
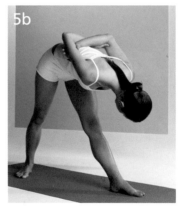

5. Warrior forward bend: From mountain pose, step back about 3–4 feet with right foot, turning right toes out 30 degrees and aligning left heel with right arch. Keep hips square, and butt, thighs, and belly tight. Bend arms behind you to grasp opposite insides of upper arms, resting forearms on lower back. Inhale while drawing spine up, keeping chest open and shoulders down (a). Exhale while bending forward from hips, drawing chest toward front thigh, and bending front leg slightly if necessary (b). Inhale and lift yourself back up, using the strength of your legs for stability. Return to mountain pose and repeat on opposite side.

yoga and pilates

The Energy-Calming Routine

Do poses 6–9 in the order listed, holding each for 4–6 breaths, using your exhalation to take you deeper into the posture.

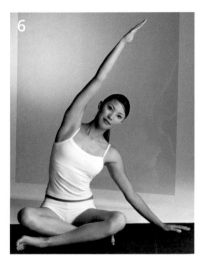

6. Seated side bend: Sitting tall with legs crossed, place fingertips on the floor at sides, arms straight and middle fingers aligned with shoulders. Keeping hips on the floor, inhale and extend right arm straight up. Exhale and walk left hand out along the floor away from left hip as you bend to the side and bring right arm overhead to the left (as shown). Hold this position, then inhale as you lift back to center while lowering right arm, and repeat on opposite side.

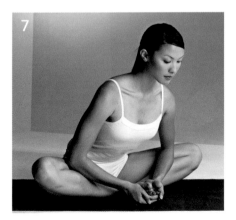

7. Butterfly: Sitting tall, place soles of feet together and as close to groin as possible, keeping torso upright. Interlace fingers under feet and let knees fall open naturally. Inhale, then exhale, leaning gently forward from hips with outside edges of feet still touching slightly and shoulders relaxed (as shown). Hold, then inhale as you lift back to center.

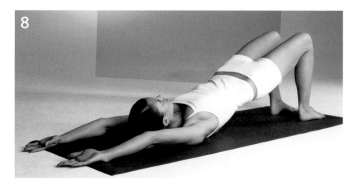

8. Moving bridge: Lie faceup on the floor with knees bent and aligned over ankles, feet hip-width apart and flat, arms relaxed on the floor alongside torso, and palms down. Inhale while extending arms overhead with palms up. Lift torso to form a straight line from shoulders to knees with shoulder blades still in contact with the floor (as shown). Exhale while lowering arms and torso to starting position and repeat 6–8 times. Hold final bridge for recommended number of breaths.

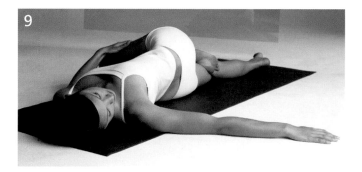

9. Spine twist: Lie faceup with legs flat on the floor, then bend right knee in toward chest, placing left hand on the outside of right knee. Extend right arm out to the side on the floor, in line with right shoulder, palm down. Inhale, then exhale while pulling right knee over left leg toward the floor; look at right hand and keep shoulders on floor (as shown). Hold position, then inhale while moving back to center position, and exhale while straightening right leg. Switch legs and repeat on opposite side.

Blast Your Ab Flab with Yoga and Pilates

What do yoga, Pilates, and wriggling into a pair of formfitting jeans have in common? They all require that you "zip" up your abs, pulling your belly in and keeping it there. With this challenging workout—a combination of some of the best yoga and Pilates moves that you can do to tighten and tone your torso—you'll soon fit into those tight pants more easily.

"Most yoga and Pilates moves force your abs to work as stabilizers," says Lisa Wheeler, a Reebok University Master Trainer based in New York City, who co-developed Reebok's Core Pilates program and who designed this workout. Using your body weight as resistance, these moves target your abs from several different angles.

Give the plan a try and you'll see amazing head-to-toe results in just 6–8 weeks—at which point you should find that zipping up your jeans has never been easier!

Guidelines: Do this workout 2–4 days a week. Perform 1 set of the (a) and (b) portions of each move in the order listed. After 6 weeks, or when you're ready, incorporate the (c) portion into your workout. Each move lists the specific number of reps that you should do.

Warm-up: Begin with the Full Sun Breaths warm-up in the previous routine to help you focus and practice moving with your breath.

Cooldown: Follow the moves with a full-body stretch: Lie on your back with legs straight and arms extended overhead, stretching hands and feet as far apart as possible. Pull knees into chest, hug them, and roll into a ball. Repeat stretch and roll 3–5 times. Then relax for as long as you like in corpse pose: Lie on your back, letting feet fall open, arms relaxed by your sides, palms up. Breathe deeply, inhaling and exhaling through nose, bringing breath to the deepest part of belly and expanding and contracting rib cage with each breath.

What you need: A sticky mat or nonslippery surface and a Reebok Core Board (page 153) for some of the Challenge moves.

Cardio and strength training: Do this as part of a program that also includes 2 days of total-body strength training and at least 3 days of cardio.

Form Facts

Practice the following techniques with each pose to achieve maximum results.

- **Align:** Make small adjustments and reposition your body as you move in and out of poses. For example, with dolphin vinyasa (4), while in forearm-plank pose (4a), shift your weight forward and backward slightly until your body is centered between your hands and feet. This will help you maintain a neutral spine.

- **Stabilize:** Pull your abs in and maintain the contraction throughout each pose to prevent your pelvis from wobbling. Draw your shoulder blades down to maintain a strong upper-torso position.

- **Extend:** Lengthen all of your limbs fully throughout each movement or position to challenge your posture and balance and to use more muscles. For example, when straightening your legs in cancan or crisscross, imagine reaching your toes as far away from you as possible, as if you're reaching out to touch an imaginary wall.

The Ab Moves

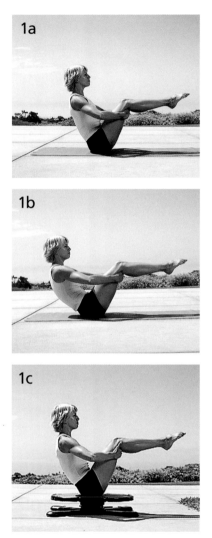

1. Boat pose (yoga): Sit erect on your "sit" bones with knees bent, feet flat on the ground, and legs and ankles squeezed together. Place hands behind the backs of thighs and lift feet up so that calves are parallel to ground (a). Hold pose for 3–5 full breaths, keeping back straight. Maintaining this position, contract abs and round spine to lower torso a few inches back toward the ground, still holding backs of thighs (b). Inhale, straighten spine, and sit back up while keeping feet raised. Repeat 3–5 times, then lower feet to ground.

The Challenge: Perform pose seated on a Reebok Core Board (c).

2a

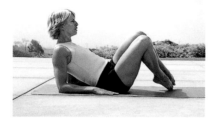

2b

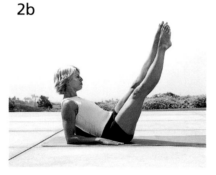

2c

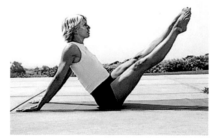

   2. Cancan (Pilates): Sit on the ground and lean back, placing forearms and hands flat on the ground with elbows under shoulders, knees bent, toes barely touching the ground, and legs and ankles together. Keeping legs together and maintaining abdominal contraction, inhale and let knees drop down to the right, toward the ground (a). Exhale and straighten legs on a diagonal (b). Inhale and bend knees (still on diagonal). Exhale, bring legs back to the center, and immediately drop them to the left, then extend on a diagonal. Continue to alternate for 8–10 reps (1 rep equals performing the move once on each side).

   The Challenge: Sit with arms extended behind you, palms on ground and fingers pointed back (c).

3a

3b

3c

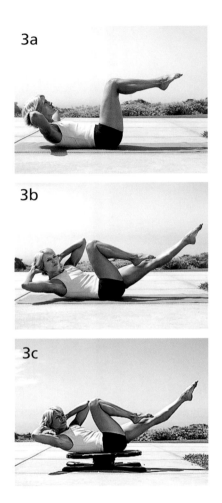

3. Crisscross (Pilates): Lie faceup with knees bent and in line with hips, calves parallel to the ground, hands behind head, fingers unclasped, and elbows open. Contract abs so that back is in contact with the ground and lift head, neck, and shoulder blades up (a). Inhale, then exhale while extending left leg at a 45-degree angle to the ground (or lower), keeping back in full contact with the ground. At the same time, rotate upper body toward right knee, keeping elbows open and lifting shoulder blades farther off the ground (b). Inhale and return torso to center, bending left knee back to starting position and keeping torso lifted. Exhale and switch, extending right leg and rotating to the left. Continue to alternate for 8–10 reps (1 rep equals completing move once with each leg).

The Challenge: Perform move lying on a Reebok Core Board (c).

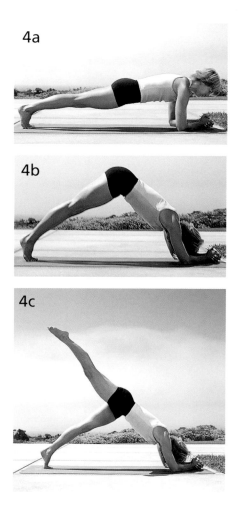

4a

4b

4c

4. Dolphin vinyasa (yoga): Kneel with forearms flat on the ground, elbows under shoulders, and knees under hips; then extend 1 leg at a time until you're supported on balls of feet, with legs and ankles together. Lower hips until body forms 1 straight line from head to heels in forearm-plank pose (a). Inhale, then exhale while pressing hips upward in dolphin pose, forming an inverted V as crown of head lowers toward ground without touching it (b). Inhale, lower to forearm-plank pose and repeat in sync with the breath. Repeat 4–6 times.

The Challenge: As you lift hips to dolphin pose, alternately extend 1 leg in the air (c), then lower leg, moving into forearm-plank pose.

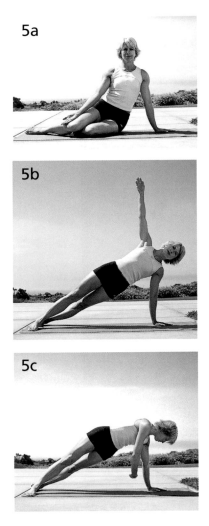

5a

5b

5c

5. Mermaid side bend (Pilates): Sit on left hip with both knees bent, left leg tucked under right, with right leg slightly extended a few inches to the right. Place left hand on the ground about 6 inches away from the body and in line with left shoulder, fingers turned outward, arm straight, and right arm resting on right knee, palm up (a). Inhale, then press down into left hand and lift hips off the ground and directly up, flexing torso to the left so that left shoulder aligns over left wrist. Extend legs and straighten arms to a T position (b). Exhale and lower to starting position, bending knees. Repeat 3–5 times on each side.

The Challenge: Stay in lifted position, then exhale and rotate torso down to face the ground, bringing right arm down and scooping underneath you (c). Inhale, rotate back up, and repeat.

The Total-Body Bonus

Yoga and Pilates aren't just great for your core muscles—these disciplines can tone your entire body. So here are 5 more moves for a total-body yoga and Pilates workout that takes you beyond the ab zone. A great adjunct to our targeted-ab workout, this series will strengthen and lengthen nearly all of your muscles.

Guidelines: Repeat the sequence of all 5 moves 4–6 times, alternating sides on the high-lunge pose each time. Do the program 2–4 times a week in conjunction with your regular strength-training and cardio workout, either on its own or along with the ab moves from earlier in this chapter.

Warm-up: Begin with the Full-Sun Breaths (page 163).

Cooldown: Finish with a full-body stretch: Lie on your back with legs straight and arms extended overhead, stretching hands and feet as far apart as possible. Pull knees into chest, hug them, and roll into a ball. Repeat stretch and roll 3–5 times. Then relax for as long as you like in corpse pose: Lie on your back and let feet fall open, arms relaxed by your sides, and palms up. Breathe deeply, inhaling and exhaling through the nose, allowing breath to reach the deepest part of belly, expanding and contracting rib cage with each breath.

The Moves

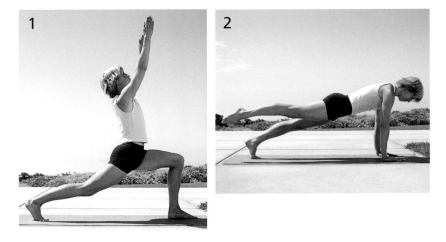

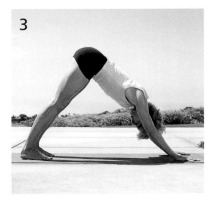

1. High lunge (yoga): Stand with legs straight, feet together, and arms by sides; then step back with right foot, bending both knees so that left knee aligns with left ankle, right leg is extended, and heel is lifted. Inhale while lifting both arms overhead (as shown). Hold for 2 breaths.

2. Leg pull-down (Pilates): From high lunge, exhale and bend forward from hips, placing hand on either side of left foot, arms straight, and wrists in line with shoulders. Step back with left foot, balancing on balls of feet, then lower hips until body forms a straight line from head to heels. Inhale and lift 1 leg to hip height (as shown). Exhale and lower leg, then inhale and lift other leg to hip height. Alternate leg lifts for 8–10 reps on each side.

3. Downward-facing dog (yoga): From leg pull-down, inhale and then exhale while lifting hips up to form an inverted V, pressing heels toward the ground. Extend spine by pressing thighs back, chest down, and chin toward chest. Draw shoulder blades back and down; rotate arms so that insides of forearms face each other (as shown). Hold for 2 breaths.

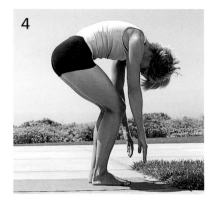

4. Standing roll-up (Pilates): From downward-facing dog, inhale, look ahead, and step 1 foot forward, then the other to bring legs and feet together with hands still on ground and knees slightly bent. Inhale, then exhale while pulling navel in toward spine as you slowly roll up to standing position (as shown), stacking shoulders over hips.

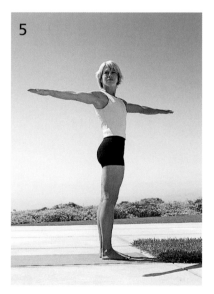

5. Standing twist (Pilates): From standing roll-up, extend both arms out to sides at shoulder height, palms down. Inhale, then exhale while contracting abs and rotating torso to right (as shown), keeping arms lifted and hips square. Inhale while rotating back to center, and exhale while rotating torso to left. Continue to alternate twists for 6–8 reps on each side.

Total-Body Power Yoga

What you might not know about yoga is that it can be a supereffective workout to burn fat and sculpt your muscles—so says *Shape* fitness editor Teri Hanson, certified trainer and "Yoga Combo" instructor in Woodland Hills, California, who designed this program, which is based on her popular class.

"You're using virtually every muscle in your body—and because you're flowing from one pose to the next you build strength *and* burn calories," Hanson explains.

An intense, hour-long yoga session burns about 455 calories (based on a 145-pound woman), which is equivalent to an hour on the elliptical trainer or inline skating. Studies done by the University of California, Davis, and Ball State University in Muncie, Indiana, have shown that yoga has cardiovascular benefits as well. Follow this plan, and you'll get a sleek and sculpted body—even if you can't make it to the gym.

Guidelines: Do this workout 2–4 days a week.

Warm-up: Begin with the Sun Salutation. Repeat the entire sequence 4–6 times.

Cooldown: From the final seated pose, roll down onto back, pull knees to chest, and rock from side to side. Then extend legs and lie flat on back in corpse pose: Lie on back, letting feet fall open, arms relaxed at sides, and palms up. Breathe deeply, inhaling and exhaling down into belly, expanding and closing rib cage with each breath. Stay here for at least 5 minutes.

Power Rx: Kick up the calorie-blasting, body-boosting benefits of this program by doing 1 Sun Salutation in between each move. This will increase the aerobic intensity of the workout.

Cardio and strength training: You should include an additional 1–2 days of resistance training and get a total of 3–5 days of cardio each week. (**Note:** This program, if done with the Power Rx, qualifies as a cardio workout.)

Her Ultimate Turning Point

Christy Turlington began modeling at age 14 and became a superstar in that world. But she frankly admits that for many years she felt uncomfortable with her own body, and her profession couldn't bring her the personal fulfillment she craved. That's one of the main reasons why she took up yoga.

Christy credits yoga with helping calm her mind enough for her to recognize her unlimited potential. She also believes that the long-sought confidence in herself and her body that it provided are what helped her kick an addiction to cigarettes. When she quit smoking, Christy gained about ten pounds—something she says met with a "cool reception" from the fashion industry. But by then, she felt good about her body and her health. Quitting smoking, along with practicing yoga, helped Christy tap in to how her body felt and to appreciate it.

"To me, the weight gain was completely worth it," she says. "I learned to accept my body exactly as it was."

Her Best Tip: Every woman has her own unique set of physical attributes that she can—and should—feel good about. "You just have to ask yourself what's right for you," says Christy. "You know when you feel your best." Practicing yoga may help you achieve that level of consciousness.

Sun Salutation Moves

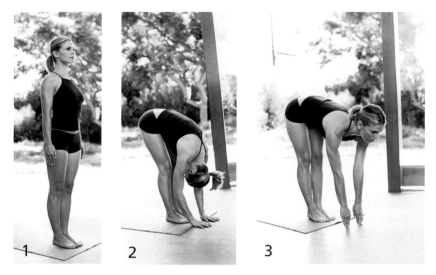

Start in mountain pose. Stand with big toes together, heels slightly apart, and legs straight (1). Place thumbs against breastbone with palms together and elbows bent. Draw shoulder blades down, tighten thigh muscles, and pull belly in, with tailbone pointing toward floor. Exhale, "hinging" forward at hip to a forward bend, with arms and head hanging toward the floor, legs straight or slightly bent, and hands touching floor (2). Inhale and look forward with fingertips still touching the floor, elongating spine and arms so that both are straight in spine prep (3).

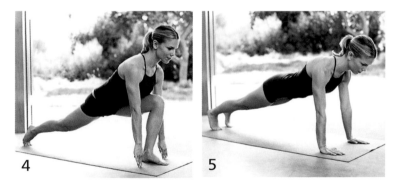

Exhale and step back with right foot into a lunge (4). Inhale while in lunge, bringing torso upright, then raise arms straight overhead. Exhale while bending forward and placing hands flat on the floor, one on each side of left foot. Inhale and step back with left foot to place feet together in plank pose (5).

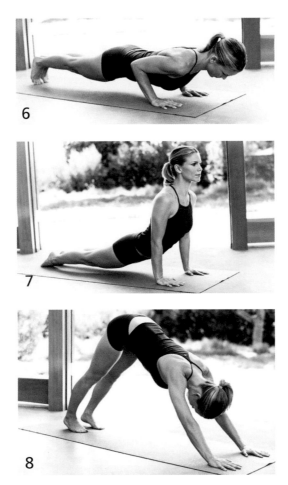

Exhale and lower torso to hover just above the floor with elbows close to side in a yogi push-up (6). Now inhale, pressing torso up into a mild back extension with elbows slightly bent. Place tops of feet on the floor, moving into upward-facing dog (7). Tuck toes under and go onto the balls of your feet, then exhale and lift hips up to downward-facing dog (8).

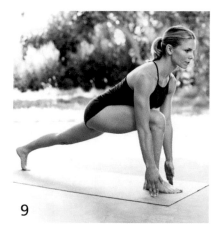

9

Inhale, stepping right leg forward into lunge (9), then raise torso to upright position with arms straight overhead.

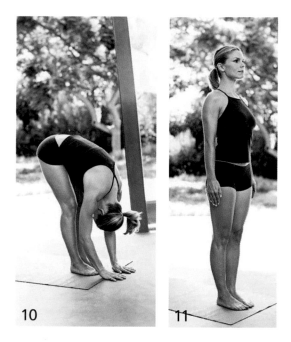

10   11

Exhale, bring hands to the floor, one on each side of right foot; then inhale while stepping left leg forward, feet together and legs straight or slightly bent in forward bend (10). Inhale, lifting torso and sweeping arms back up overhead; then exhale while lowering arms to sides again in mountain pose (11).

The Yoga Power Moves

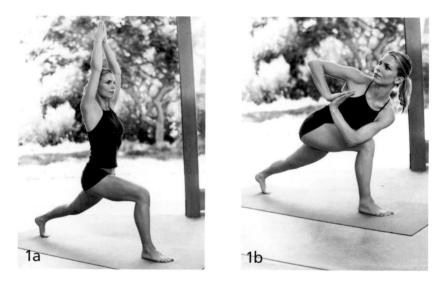

1a

1b

1. Revolving crescent: From mountain pose, step back with left foot, bending right knee to align with right ankle, keeping left knee slightly bent and heel lifted. Inhale, extending arms overhead with palms together (a). Exhale, hinging at hips and rotating torso to right, placing left elbow on the outside of right thigh. With palms still pressed together, look back past right elbow (b). Hold the rotation for 3–5 breaths. Inhale, bringing torso to an upright position with legs still in lunge while extending arms overhead (a). Exhale while lowering arms to sides, and step feet together, lifting torso and sweeping arms overhead, then down to mountain pose. Switch legs and repeat on opposite side. Repeat sequence once more on each side.

Power Rx: Do one full Sun Salutation before continuing to next move.

Strengthens the entire core of the body, firming legs, hips, and butt while improving overall balance and control.

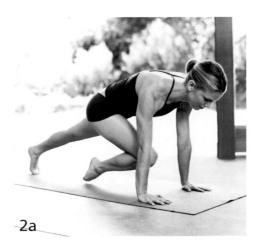

2a

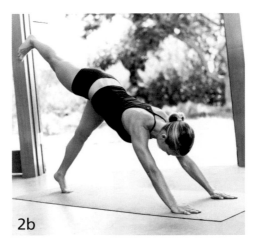

2b

2. Plank to leg extension: From mountain pose, inhale and sweep arms overhead, then exhale while going into a forward bend. Step feet back to plank pose, body forming a straight line from head to heels. Lift right leg to hip height. Inhale, then exhale while bending right knee in toward chest (a). Inhale while extending right leg behind you, pressing hips upward, and continuing to lift leg (b). Exhale, lowering leg and hips, and repeat knee pull and leg extension 4–6 times.

After final rep, swing right leg forward to place foot on the floor between hands. Bring feet together into forward bend. Inhale, lifting torso and sweeping arms overhead, then exhale while lowering arms to mountain pose. Switch legs and repeat. Perform sequence once more on each side.

Power Rx: Do one full Sun Salutation before continuing to next move.
Increases strength, stamina, and flexibility while creating a sense of grace.

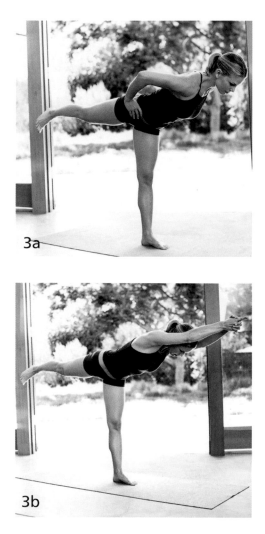

3a

3b

3. Warrior III: From mountain pose, place hands on hips and extend right leg behind you, with toes lightly touching floor, leg straight, left knee slightly bent, and torso upright with shoulders and hips square. Inhale, then exhale while bending forward from hips until torso is parallel to floor, bringing right leg even higher so that it aligns with torso (a). If you can keep your balance, extend both arms forward in line with torso, fingers interlaced and index fingers pointing forward (b). Hold for 3–5 breaths; then slowly stand up and place right foot back on the floor, lowering arms to return to mountain pose, and repeat on opposite side. Repeat once more on each side.

Power Rx: Do one full Sun Salutation before continuing to next move.

Strengthens the legs, hips, and spine while improving balance and concentration, which will give you a sense of empowerment.

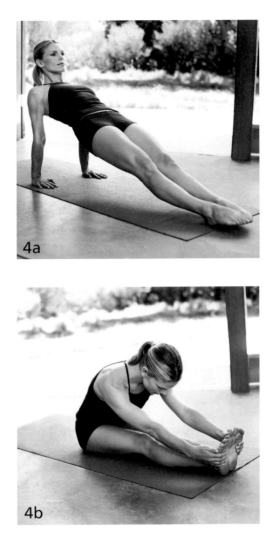

4. Plank to forward bend: Sit on a mat with torso erect, legs extended, feet together and gently flexed, hands by hips, and arms straight. Inhale and lift yourself off the mat as a single unit so that you're balancing on hand and heels, body forming a line from shoulders to heels and toes pointed (a). Exhale and lower hips to the mat to sit. Inhale while lifting both arms overhead; then exhale and hinge forward into a seated forward bend while reaching hands toward feet with arms straight, and feet flexed (b). Inhale, sweeping arms overhead while returning to upright seated position. Exhale and lower arms to sides. Repeat sequence 4–6 times.

Strengthens and stretches the entire body in perfect balance, but also has a calming effect and brings a sense of completion to your workout.

Ultimate Word

Practicing yoga at home might encourage you to look for a class. That can be a confusing process since you'll see classes listed under a variety of names. Hatha yoga is the most widely practiced form of physical yoga in the United States, under which many other types are grouped. Some of the popular hatha derivatives, such as ashtanga and viniyoga, are movement and breath oriented and can offer a significant challenge. Iyengar strives for precise form, using props like chairs or blocks and holding positions for longer periods of time. Bikram, also known as "hot yoga," encompasses a demanding, set sequence in a 90-degree-plus room. (Use caution and drink plenty of water if you do Bikram.) Forms such as kundalini and tantra focus on energy, breath work, and stress release more than on the postures themselves.

You might also want to try a Pilates class. These exercises were originally designed to be done on a machine called a Reformer. Reformer classes are widely available, but since they're often held on an individual basis or in small groups, they can be pricey. These days, most gyms have mat Pilates classes, where you perform the same moves but use simple equipment such as rubber tubing and resistance circles (or no equipment at all).

To supplement all these routines, we've recommended 3–5 days of cardio each week, and our next chapter will give you a variety of heart-healthy programs to choose from.

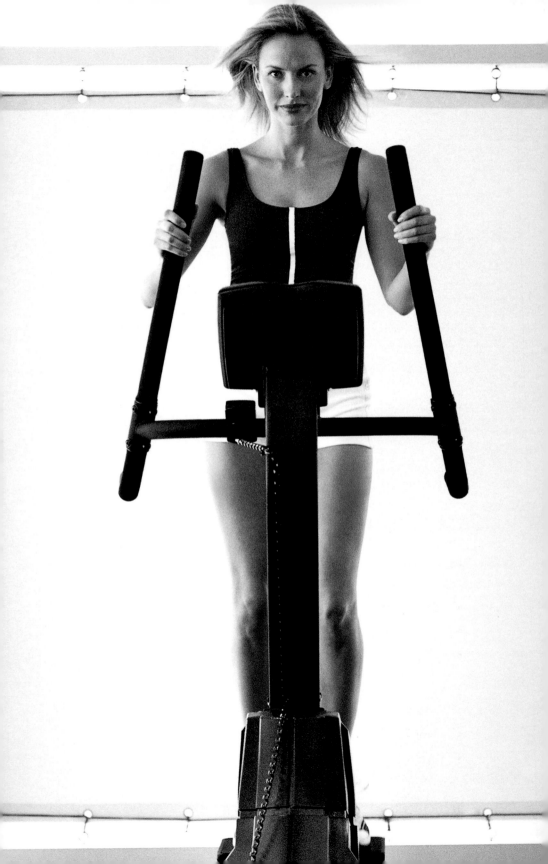

chapter 9

fat-burning
(and tush-toning)
cardio

Cardio exercise is a vital component of overall fitness, and you won't achieve a trim, strong body without including it in your regimen. It can also help ensure that you stay healthy by reducing your risk for heart disease, diabetes, high blood pressure, and some types of cancer. And there's nothing quite like a vigorous, blood-pumping workout to make your skin glow, lift your mood, and put a smile on your face.

This Chapter's To-Do List

In the following pages, you'll learn:

- Some common cardio myths

- How much of this training you should do

- Complete plans for trimming down, having more energy, and getting a gorgeous lower body

- More effective training techniques to help you reach your goals

- Tips for boosting your intensity and metabolism

- Ways to incorporate cardio with your strength training for a more sculpted body

Do You Have a (Cardio) Clue?

Some of you might already be cardio junkies—running, Spinning, stepping, kickboxing, or swimming—but are you maximizing your benefits? And those of you who are new to doing aerobic exercise may have some misconceptions about the best ways to go about it. Do you know the secret to blasting fat and getting in better shape? Is it:

- Superlong or extremely difficult aerobic workouts?
- Exercising every day?
- Using one particular machine?
- Keeping your heart rate in the "fat-burning zone"?

Start by taking our quiz to find out what you do and don't know about the secrets to cardio success. Answer the following questions "true" or "false."

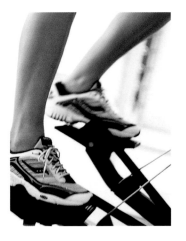

1. For maximum fat loss, you should keep your heart rate in the "fat-burning zone."

False. It's a myth that you'll burn more fat by keeping your heart rate low, says certified trainer Paul Robbins, at the elite training center Athletes Performance in Tempe, Arizona. When you exercise at a lower intensity, a high percentage of your fuel comes from fat versus carbohydrates—but you're burning fewer calories overall, which means that your waistline loses out. "Total calories burned is always more important than what kind of fuel you're burning," he says. And you can burn more calories by working out at a higher, not lower, intensity.

2. You can build all the lower-body strength you need from cardio workouts like running and stair climbing.

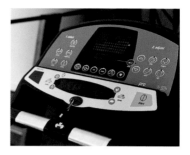

False. Weight-bearing aerobic activities can strengthen your lower body to a degree. But to really develop muscle, prevent injury, and shape your lower body, it's important to do strength exercises that work your legs and glutes in more than one repetitive movement pattern. By strength training, you can also make your cardio workouts more productive. "The stronger your lower body is, the harder and longer you'll be able to train," Robbins explains. That translates to more calories burned and more visible results.

3. Some cardio machines are better than others when it comes to getting a great aerobic workout.

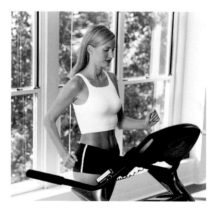

False. You can get just as good of a workout whether you're using a treadmill, an elliptical trainer, or a rowing machine. The caveat: Some people may not work as hard on one machine as another, so be sure to work at a high enough intensity to get your heart rate up. Robbins recommends choosing the manual setting and plugging in your own program rather than relying on a preset workout that may or not push you hard enough. He also suggests choosing equipment that works both your upper and lower body at once, such as cross-country skiing and rowing machines.

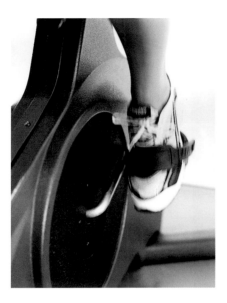

4. If you're not tired and dripping with sweat by the end of your workout, you haven't pushed yourself hard enough.

False. A good cardio workout should leave you feeling energized, not lethargic. If you're exhausted afterward, you've pushed too hard. And while sweat can be an indication of how hard you're working, it isn't always. "The amount of sweat a person produces often has more to do with core body temperature, air temperature, and genetics than her level of exertion," Robbins explains.

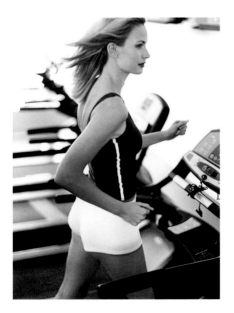

5. Longer workouts burn more calories.

False. You can actually expend more calories in less time by doing shorter, more intense interval work-outs. By getting your heart rate up, you not only burn a lot of calories, but you also boost your metabolic rate, so your body continues burning extra calories for up to several hours after you're finished.

6. You need to do 6–7 high-intensity aerobic work-outs a week in order to build optimal cardiovascular strength and endurance.

False. You can't exercise intensely every day, because that will lead to injury and burnout. Adequate rest is necessary for muscle recovery and can improve the quality of your workouts. Do no more than 2 or 3 high-intensity cardio sessions in a week, alternating with moderate- or lower-intensity workouts.

Your Cardio Guidelines

We've just given you a lot of what *not* to do. So exactly how should you fit cardio into your workout regimen? That depends on your goals.

- **To maintain your health,** get a total of 30 minutes of moderate to vigorous physical activity almost daily. This should be over and above your usual going-about-your-business activity.

- **For fitness,** ratchet up to doing aerobic exercise 3–5 days a week for 20–60 minutes at 60–90 percent of your maximum heart rate (MHR). The most popular way to calculate MHR is to simply subtract your age from 220, but this tends to overestimate in younger people and underestimate it in the over-40 group. To get a better idea of your actual MHR, follow this formula: 208 – (0.7 x your age) = MHR.

- **To lose weight and keep it off,** you may need 60–90 minutes of at least moderate-intensity activity most days of the week.

To help you put these guiding principles into action, we've devised three cardio programs for you to choose from, depending on your goals:

1. A smart all-around cardio/strength regimen to promote good health.

2. A running or walking fat-burning program that shows results in just six weeks.

3. A program using cardio machines that emphasizes tightening and toning your tush.

At the end of the chapter are some stretches to do after whichever program you choose.

Her Ultimate Turning Point

For as long as she could remember, Mickey Messina of Pennsylvania was heavier than her peers. But it wasn't until she was in junior high that she determined to do something about her weight. Many of her friends were dating, while her 185-pound body was keeping her from enjoying her teenage years.

"I started by doing some form of exercise at the gym regularly," she says. "At first, I walked on the treadmill, but once I attended a step-aerobics class, I was hooked." Once that became a habit, she added strength training and healthy eating. She began seeing changes in just a month, and after two years had lost 75 pounds and fit into size-6 clothes.

Her Best Tip: In order to commit to a routine, remind yourself of all the positive aspects of working out (including how good you feel afterward).

1. Smart-Cardio Workout

In this program, you'll do 3 cardio workouts a week—2 endurance (steady-state) and one power (interval) to boost your heart strength and improve your overall fitness. You can use any cardio machine, or get outside and run or walk; for the best results, try to vary your activities throughout the week.

You'll also do 2 lower-body strength-training workouts a week on the same days as your cardio-endurance sessions, to help you muscle through your cardio and reduce your risk of injury.

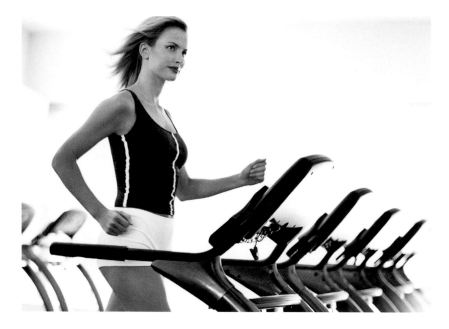

Warm-up/cooldown: On your strength-training/cardio-endur-ance days: Do 5 minutes of lower-intensity cardio, any activity of your choice, before your strength workout. On all days: At the end of your workout, stretch your lower body, holding each stretch for 20–30 seconds without bouncing, and repeat 3–5 times.

Your workout week at-a-glance: Use the Rate of Perceived Exertion (RPE) to gauge your intensity during aerobic exercise. If you want to do more than 3 cardio workouts per week, you can include 1–2 additional days of lower-intensity activity (such as walking, light hiking, cycling, or power yoga), as long as it's not too taxing on your legs. Be sure to take at least 1 full day off per week.

Rate of Perceived Exertion (RPE)

You'll get the best results if you work at the designated intensity for each session. Monitor it using this key.

RPE 1–2   Very easy; you can converse with no effort.

RPE 3:   Easy; you can converse with almost no effort.

RPE 4:   Moderately easy; you can converse comfortably with little effort.

RPE 5:   Moderate; conversation requires some effort.

RPE 6:   Moderately difficult; conversation requires quite a bit of effort.

RPE 7:   Difficult; conversation requires a lot of effort.

RPE 8:   Very difficult; conversation requires maximum effort.

RPE 9–10: Peak effort; no-talking zone.

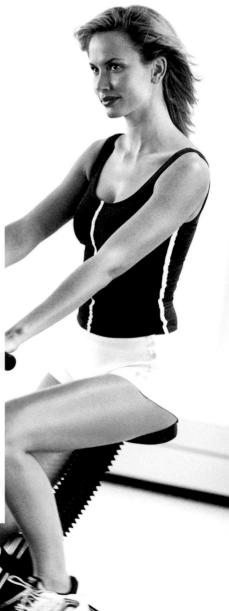

Here's an example of how your week might look:

MON: Lower-body strengthener moves,
plus cardio-endurance workout

TUES: *Optional:* Low-intensity cardio such as
walking, light hiking, cycling, or power yoga

WED: Cardio-power workout

THU: Rest

FRI: Lower-body strengthener moves,
plus cardio-endurance workout

SAT: *Optional:* Low-intensity cardio such as
walking, light hiking, cycling, or power yoga

SUN: Rest

Cardio-Endurance Workout

Goal: You'll boost cardiovascular fitness and work at a fairly high intensity for long bouts, which will increase stamina and burn calories.

Game plan: In this workout, you'll do two 10-minute, mostly steady-state bouts with small fluctuations in intensity. By varying your intensity slightly, you'll be able to work harder longer and use more lower-body muscles for better overall toning.

Frequency: Twice a week, *after* your lower-body strengthener workout.

To progress: Before your cooldown, add an additional 8:2 interval (8 minutes at a steady intensity and 2 minutes at a step-down intensity, for 10 minutes total) every 6 weeks, building up to a total workout time of 60 minutes.

Workout	Time	RPE
Warm-up	5 min.	4
Steady intensity	8 min.	6–7
Step-down	2 min.	4–5
Steady intensity	8 min.	6–7
Step-down	2 min.	4–5
Cool-down	5 min.	3
TOTAL TIME	30 min.	

Calories Burned: 288 (plus 110 for each additional 10-minute interval), based upon a 145-pound woman.

Cardio-Power Workout

Goal: You'll boost cardiovascular strength and speed by increasing your ability to train at a high intensity, which translates into an elevated metabolism and more calories burned during and after your workout.

Game plan: In this interval workout, you'll be alternating short bouts of high- and low-intensity work. By pushing your body and then allowing it to recover, you can boost your heart rate in a not-too-strenuous manner.

Frequency: Once a week.

To progress: Add an additional 2:2 (4 minutes total) interval to your workout every 4–6 weeks (not to exceed a total workout time of 60 minutes).

Workout	Time	RPE
Warm-up	5 min.	4
Moderate push	2 min.	6
High push	2 min.	7–8
Moderate push	2 min.	6
High push	2 min.	7–8
Moderate push	2 min.	6
High push	2 min.	7–8
Moderate push	2 min.	6
High push	2 min.	7–8
Moderate push	2 min.	6
High push	2 min.	7–8
Cool-down	5 min.	3
TOTAL TIME	30 min.	

Calories Burned: 307 (plus 48 for each additional 4-minute interval), based upon a 145-pound woman.

Q. Should you do your cardio workouts in the morning so that you'll tap in to your stored fat instead of using the calories and fat you ate throughout the day?

A. "There is no advantage either way," says Glenn Gaesser, Ph.D., director of the kinesiology program at the University of Virginia in Charlottesville. "It's the total-calorie balance over 24 hours that's critical." In other words, if you burn more calories than you consume—whether you're jogging in front of the *Today* show or *The Tonight Show*—you'll lose weight. Conversely, if you eat more calories than your body burns, you'll end up gaining.

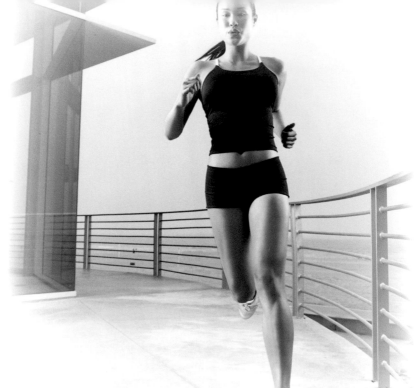

Lower-Body Strengtheners

Adding lower-body strength training to your cardio program 2 days a week will give you the kind of power and strength you need for optimal aerobic performance. The primary and stabilizing muscles in your lower body, as well as your core (abdominals and back extensors) will be stronger and more balanced, as will your hips, knees, and shins. You'll also increase stride length and improve push-off strength, both of which are especially important for cardio activities such as walking and running. If you're doing some of the moves in the thigh and upper-body workouts, plan them for these days. Otherwise, incorporate these exercises into your program.

Details: Do 2 sets (12 reps each) of the first 3 strength-training exercises in the order listed, followed by the 3- to 5-minute heel walk. Perform these moves prior to your cardio-endurance workout, because doing cardio after weight training can help flush the lactic acid from your muscles. Use as much weight as you can (where applicable), and complete all sets and reps with good form. Rest 30–60 seconds between sets.

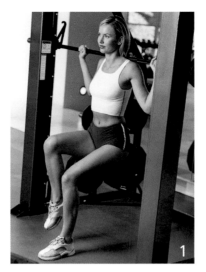

1. Smith machine one-legged squat: Stand inside a Smith machine, bar resting on shoulders, hands slightly more than shoulder-width apart, palms forward, elbows pointing down, and feet slightly ahead of bar. Keeping abs contracted, chest lifted, and torso erect, unlock bar and lift right foot with right knee bent. Bend left knee and sit back onto left heel with back aligned under bar (lower back naturally curved), and lower yourself into squat position (as shown). Contract buttocks as you straighten left knee to starting position. Repeat for 1 set of reps, then switch legs and repeat.

Starting weight: Up to 20 pounds per side, depending on machine.

Strengthens hamstrings, quadriceps, buttocks, and calves; abductors and adductors act as stabilizers.

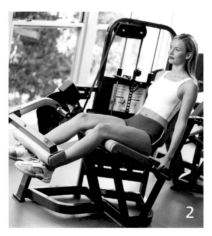

2. Leg-extension combos: Sit with hips and back against back pad, with roller pad adjusted to ankle height and lower legs hanging, knees bent at 90 degrees; hold support handles. Contract abs, then press roller up and out until legs are extended straight. Lower halfway down (as shown), then press up and straighten legs again before lowering to starting position. Each portion of the move should take 2 counts, for a total of 8 counts per rep.

Starting weight: 20–35 pounds.

Strengthens quadriceps with emphasis on the medial portion.

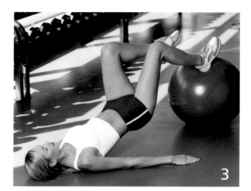

3. One-legged bridge ham curl: Lie faceup on floor and place heels hip-width apart on top of a stability ball with legs straight and arms by sides. Press right heel into ball, then raise left knee, bent in line with hip, so calf is parallel to floor. Contract abs, then lift hips up into a bridge so that body forms a straight line from shoulders to ankles; at the same time, roll ball toward hips, pulling with right heel (as shown). As you make the bridge, shift weight only onto shoulders, not onto neck. Pause at top of lift, then slowly lower to starting position as you roll ball away from you with right heel, keeping hips level. Complete all reps, then switch legs.

Note: If this move is too challenging, do the same exercise with both heels on the ball, hip-width apart or closer (the closer your feet, the harder the move), pulling with both heels.

Strengthens hamstrings and buttocks; improves core strength.

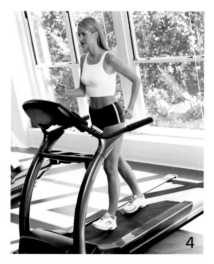

4. Heel walk: Set a treadmill at a 0 percent grade and choose a pace that allows you to walk at a comfortable stride (about 3–3.5 mph), so you're not leaning forward or backward. Maintain an upright torso and look straight ahead (as shown). Keeping the balls of both feet lifted, walk for 3–5 minutes, changing the incline as follows: Do 1–2 minutes at 0 percent incline, 30 seconds–1 minute at 1 percent incline, 30 seconds–1 minute at 2 percent incline, and 30 seconds–1 minute at 0 percent. (For your first week, start with 3 minutes, gradually adding time until you're up to 5.)

Strengthens shins and stretches calves.

Misstep:

Letting hot or cold weather quash your exercise plans. Instead, think of it as an opportunity to expand your fitness horizons as well as your abilities. "Unless you're training for an event, use the opportunity to make your muscles move differently," suggests Annette Lang, a Reebok University Master Trainer in New York City. You'll boost your fitness and maybe even improve your performance in your favorite activity when the weather gets better. Just be sure to get proper instruction before you try something brand-new.

Here are some fun, effective indoor alternatives to outdoor workouts: Instead of walking or hiking, do step aerobics; try Spinning in place of bicycling or running; replace in-line skating with balance-board moves; and substitute sports-based classes such as boot camps or athletic conditioning for tennis.

2. Walk or Run Fat-Burning Workout

Losing weight can be as simple as putting one foot in front of the other. To show you how easy a slimming-down program can be for just about anyone, we sought the help of exercise physiologist Ray Browning, M.S., of Nederland, Colorado. He put together a workout featuring a walking, walking/running, or running program that requires just 15–45 minutes, 3–5 days a week. Whether you're ready for a 5K or just starting out, you'll see measurable results in about 6 weeks.

In addition to doing a strength workout of your choice twice a week, pick a walking, walking/running, or running program according to your ability level and the following guidelines:

- **The walking workout:** You're just starting out, prefer walking to running, or don't want to stress your joints.

- **The walking/running workout:** You like the variety of both walking and running; you're already walking at least 30 minutes, 3 times a week; and you want to add some running.

- **The running workout:** You're comfortable running for at least 30 minutes at an easy pace 5 times a week.

To progress: If you're currently walking and your goal is to run, begin in the 4th week of the walking workout and continue through Week 6, then progress to the walking/running workout. If you're currently doing walking/running workouts and your goal is continual running, begin with Week 4 of the walking/running workout and continue through Week 6, then begin the running workout.

Warm-up/cooldown: Start and finish each workout with 5 minutes of easy walking. Follow the cooldown walking with stretches. Hold each stretch for 20–30 seconds without bouncing and repeat 3–5 times.

Monitor Your Intensity

You'll get the best results if you work at the designated intensity for each session, using this key:

- **Easy walk or run:** 60–70 percent of your maximum heart rate (MHR); 3–4 on a scale of 1–10 where 10 is the most difficult; you should be able to maintain this level and carry on a conversation.

- **Moderately easy walk or run:** 70–75 percent of MHR; 5–6 on a scale of 1–10; you can maintain this level and exchange a few sentences at a time.

- **Moderate walk or run:** 75–80 percent of MHR; 7–8 on a scale of 1–10; conversation is limited to a few words at a time.

- **Speed walk or moderately difficult run:** 80–90 percent of MHR; 9 on a scale of 1–10; conversation is limited to one-word exchanges.

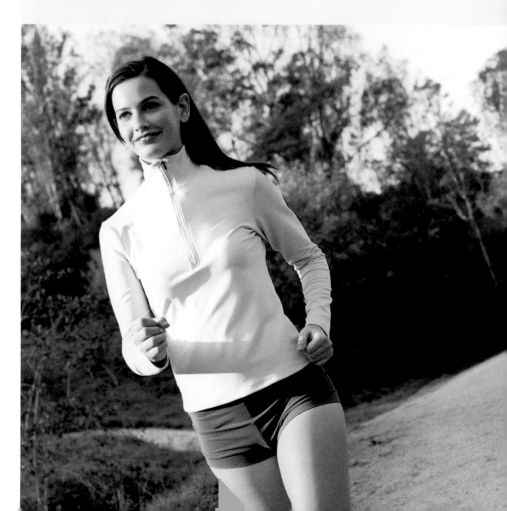

Here's your 6-week cardio calendar:

WEEK ONE

DAY 1

walking workout	15 min. easy walk
walking/running workout	25 min. easy walk
running workout	30 min. easy run

DAY 2

walking workout	15 min. moderately easy walk
walking/running workout	4 min. moderately easy walk, 1 min. moderately easy run; repeat for 20 min. total
running workout	25 min. moderately easy run

DAY 3

walking workout	20 min. easy walk
walking/running workout	30 min. easy walk
running workout	30 min. easy run

DAY 4

walking workout	OFF
walking/running workout	25 min. moderately easy walk
running workout	25 min. moderately easy run

DAY 5

walking workout	OFF
walking/running workout	OFF
running workout	25 min. moderate run

WEEK TWO

DAY 1

walking workout	20 min. easy walk
walking/running workout	30 min. easy walk
running workout	35 min. easy run

DAY 2

walking workout	15 min. moderately easy walk
walking/running workout	3 min. moderately easy walk, 2 min. moderately easy run; repeat for 25 min. total
running workout	25 min. moderate run

DAY 3

walking workout	20 min. easy walk
walking/running workout	30 min. easy walk
running workout	30 min. easy run

DAY 4

walking workout	20 min. moderately easy walk
walking/running workout	25 min. moderately easy walk
running workout	30 min. moderately easy run

DAY 5

walking workout	OFF
walking/running workout	OFF
running workout	20 min. moderate run

fat-burning cardio

WEEK THREE

DAY 1

walking workout	25 min. easy walk
walking/running workout	30 min. easy walk
running workout	40 min. easy run

DAY 2

walking workout	20 min. moderately easy walk
walking/running workout	3 min. moderately easy walk, 3 min. moderately easy run; repeat for 18–24 min. total
running workout	30 min. moderate run

DAY 3

walking workout	20 min. easy walk
walking/running workout	2 min. moderately easy walk, 2 min. moderately easy run; repeat for 24–26 min. total
running workout	30 min. moderately easy run

DAY 4

walking workout	4 min. moderately easy walk, 1 min. speed walk; repeat for 15 min. total
walking/running workout	30 min. easy walk
running workout	2 min. moderately difficult run, 1 min. easy run; repeat for 21 min. total

DAY 5

walking workout	OFF
walking/running workout	2 min. moderately easy walk, 2 min. moderately easy run repeat for 24–26 min. total
running workout	30 min. moderately easy run

WEEK FOUR

DAY 1

walking workout	30 min. easy walk
walking/running workout	35 min. easy walk
running workout	45 min. easy run

DAY 2

walking workout	25 min. moderately easy walk
walking/running workout	2 min. moderately easy walk, 3 min. moderate run; repeat for 25 min. total
running workout	30 min. moderate easy run

DAY 3

walking workout	25 min. easy walk
walking/running workout	30 min. moderately easy walk
running workout	30 min. moderately easy run

DAY 4

walking workout	4 min. moderately easy walk, 1 min. speed walk; repeat for 20 min. total
walking/running workout	30 min. easy walk
running workout	3 min. moderately difficult run, 2 min. moderately easy run; repeat for 25 min. total

DAY 5

walking workout	25 min. moderately easy walk
walking/running workout	2 min. moderately easy walk, 3 min. moderate run; repeat for 20 min. total
running workout	30 min. easy run

fat-burning cardio

WEEK FIVE

DAY 1

walking workout	30 min. easy walk
walking/running workout	40 min. easy walk
running workout	45 min. easy run

DAY 2

walking workout	3 min. moderately easy walk, 2 min. speed walk; repeat for 25 min. total
walking/running workout	2 min. moderately difficult run, 2 min. easy walk; repeat for 28–32 min. total
running workout	1 min. moderately difficult run, 1 min. easy run; repeat for 24–26 min. total

DAY 3

walking workout	30 min. easy walk
walking/running workout	30 min. moderately easy walk
running workout	30 min. moderately easy run

DAY 4

walking workout	3 min. moderately easy walk, 2 min. speed walk; repeat for 20 min. total
walking/running workout	30 min. easy walk
running workout	4 min. moderately difficult run, 1 min. easy run; repeat for 24 min. total

DAY 5

walking workout	30 min. moderately easy walk
walking/running workout	1 min. moderately easy walk, 4 min. moderate run; repeat for 25 min. total
running workout	30 min. easy run

WEEK SIX

DAY 1

walking workout	35 min. easy walk
walking/running workout	40 min. easy walk
running workout	45 min. easy run

DAY 2

walking workout	3 min. moderately easy walk, 2 min. speed walk; repeat for 25 min. total
walking/running workout	2 min. moderately difficult run, 1 min. easy walk; repeat for 24 min. total
running workout	2 min. moderately difficult run, 2 min. easy run; repeat for 28–32 min. total

DAY 3

walking workout	30 min. easy walk
walking/running workout	1 min. moderately easy walk, 1 min. moderately easy run; repeat for 30 min. total
running workout	30 min. moderately easy run

DAY 4

walking workout	2 min. moderately easy walk, 3 min. speed walk; repeat for 25 min. total
walking/running workout	30 min. easy walk
running workout	4 min. moderately difficult run, 2 min. easy run; repeat for 30 min. total

DAY 5

walking workout	30 min. moderately easy walk
walking/running workout	1 min. moderately easy walk, 5 min. moderate run; repeat for 30 min. total
running workout	30 min. easy run

Tips to Take Weight Off

- **Ramp it up.** Walking or running on an incline, or climbing steps, torches a lot more calories than going at the same intensity on a flat surface.

- **Bound.** As you walk or run, add intervals of explosive movement—leap in zigzag fashion up a trail or jump from rock to rock. You'll use more muscles to keep your balance and bound, and you'll work new muscles, too.

- **Walk with poles.** A recent study showed that using poles can burn 20–25 percent more calories. But don't just carry them; make sure that you swing, plant, and push off.

- **Change surfaces.** Grass, sand, and dirt make your work harder than pavement or concrete. (Soft sand is tops, upping calories burned by 30–50 percent.) Try interval sessions where you alternate be-tween hard and soft sand or a track and grass, keeping the pace the same.

3. Best-Butt Cardio Workout

To help his female clients achieve the ubiquitous goal of a great butt, Reebok University Master Trainer Jeffrey Scott shows them how to work the right muscles and blast fat. He created these tush-toning cardio programs so that you can get the same benefits. "Using these machines and these programs promotes the use of muscle—especially the buttocks muscles—rather than momentum, which is often not the case in other cardio workouts," Scott explains. "Plus, these plans' interval and/or progressive-intensity formats are optimal ways to burn the most calories in the shortest time."

You can mix and match the programs throughout the week, which will bust boredom, prevent a plateau, and help you avoid overuse injuries.

Guidelines: Do either of these cardio workouts 3–5 times a week using the RPE (page 198) to gauge your intensity. A warm-up and cooldown are built into each workout. End by stretching, holding each stretch for 20–30 seconds without bouncing.

Beginner option: If you're just starting out with an exercise program, try doing only 3 workouts per week. You can also cut 2–5 minutes off the workout you select (making sure to do the prescribed warm-up and cooldown).

Advanced option: If you've been working out regularly for the past 6 months, try doing your cardio workouts 5 times a week. You can also add 2–5 minutes to the workout you select (making sure to do the prescribed warm-up and cooldown).

Program 1: Treadmill Tush Toner

On the treadmill, walk tall with head up, shoulders back, and abdominals in. Always step with the heel first, rolling onto and pushing off the ball of the foot. Pump your arms to increase the calorie burn.

How it works: When you walk or run, the steeper the incline, the more you use your buttocks muscles. A slant also increases the intensity at which you're working, which dramatically ups your calorie expenditure (as long as you're maintaining the same speed). For example, a 145-pound woman walking on a level surface at 3.5 mph will burn about 300 calories an hour, but she'll blast 400 calories an hour going the same speed on a 4 percent incline and 500 calories an hour at the same speed on a 10 percent incline.

Set a treadmill on manual and perform the workout according to the chart below. We've mapped out how to raise and lower your RPE by increasing and decreasing the incline, so you'll get the maximum butt benefits.

Take it outside: Walk or run on a hilly trail or footpath. If you can't find the right hills to adjust your RPE, you can alter your intensity by simply changing your pace (though the butt benefit won't be quite as great).

Workout	Time	RPE	Incline %
Warm-up	5 min.	4	0
Steady climb	30 sec.	5	3
	30 sec.	6	6
	30 sec.	7	9
	30 sec.	8	12
Recovery	3 min.	4	0
Rise and fall	1 min.	5	3
	1 min.	6	6
	1 min.	7	9
	1 min.	8	12
	1 min.	7	9
	1 min.	6	6
	1 min.	5	3
Recovery	3 min.	4	0
Steady climb	30 sec.	5	3
	30 sec.	6	6
	30 sec.	7	9
	30 sec.	8	12
Cooldown	5 min.	4	0
TOTAL TIME	27 min.		

Calories Burned:
235, based upon a 145-pound woman

Program 2:
Stair-Climbing Supersculptor

Although you'll be angled forward slightly at the hips, don't rest on the stair-climber's rails. Keep chest lifted, abdominals tight, and hands lightly touching the rails or at sides. Lower the intensity if your form is being sacrificed.

How it works: A stair-climber effectively sculpts the hamstrings and buttocks muscles, since they work through a full range of motion as you lift your knees up higher and push through the heels as you step. Meanwhile, the interval format of this program enables you to burn more calories in less time so that you'll blast away that extra flab.

Set a stair-climber on manual and perform the workout according to the chart below. You can adjust your intensity by speeding up (which actually requires *lowering* the resistance) or slowing down (which requires *upping* the resistance), as dictated by the applicable RPE.

Take it outside: Find a hiking trail with rolling hills and rocky terrain, preferably one that has increasingly steep inclines, separated by flat surfaces for recovery. Since hiking requires a similar range of motion to that of a stair-climber, it's a great outdoor butt and thigh burner.

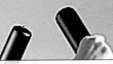

Workout	Time	RPE
Warm-up	5 min.	4
Interval 1	30 sec.	6
	30 sec.	7
	30 sec.	8
	30 sec.	9
Recovery	2 min.	4
Interval 2	1 min.	5
	1 min.	6
	1 min.	7
	1 min.	8
Recovery	2 min.	4
Interval 3	30 sec.	6
	30 sec.	7
	30 sec.	8
	30 sec.	9
Recovery	2 min.	4
Interval 4	1 min.	5
	1 min.	6
	1 min.	7
	1 min.	8
Cooldown	4 min.	4
TOTAL TIME	27 min.	

Calories Burned:
235, based upon a 145-pound woman

Jump for Joy

Boxers do it and so do little girls
. . . but how does jumping rope
rate as a cardio activity? "It can
develop nearly every area of fitness,
including aerobic fitness, anaerobic
fitness, speed, agility, coordination,
timing, rhythm, and muscular
endurance," says Leigh Crews, a
spokeswoman for the American
Council on Exercise and a certified
trainer in Rome, Georgia.

"Jumping rope is an excellent
activity for weight loss if you follow
some basic precautions," she says.
To minimize the impact on your
joints, Crews advises that you bend
your knees slightly as you land, and
jump only high enough to clear
the rope. Also, try to work on a
shock-absorbent surface such as
rubberized flooring or hardwood
(although padded carpet or dirt will
do); grass is also fine but tends to
catch the rope. Avoid jumping on
asphalt and concrete, which don't
absorb the shock.

Even if you're already fit,
jumping rope can quickly leave you
breathless, and your calf muscles
will likely feel sore afterward, so
start by doing intervals. Alternate
30 consecutive jumps with about 30
seconds of walking in place. As you
walk, hold both ends of the

rope in one hand and swing it in a figure-eight motion at your side. Gradually increase the length of your jumping intervals to the point where you can jump for several minutes at a time. Cut yourself some slack if you're tripping over your feet—this is a skill that has to be developed.

Once you've relearned your grade-school technique, you'll find that jumping rope burns a tremendous number of calories. A 145-pound woman can burn about 174 calories in 15 minutes (by comparison, walking a 15-minute-per-mile pace burns about 78 calories). Still, to lose weight, you generally need to burn more calories than that per day, so Crews recommends combining this with other cardio activities rather than jumping for longer periods. And if you experience knee strain, even after building up gradually, try a different activity.

The Stretch Moves

Whichever cardio program you choose, always do these lower-body stretches after your cooldown, according the instructions in the workouts.

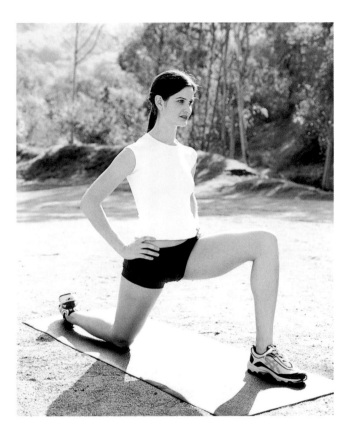

1. Quadriceps stretch: Kneel with right knee, shin, and top of right foot on the ground; left leg bent with ankle in front of knee; and hands on hips. Keeping torso upright and abs contracted, press hips forward gently until you feel a stretch in the front of the right hip and thigh, moving left knee over left ankle (as shown). Release and complete all reps, then switch legs.

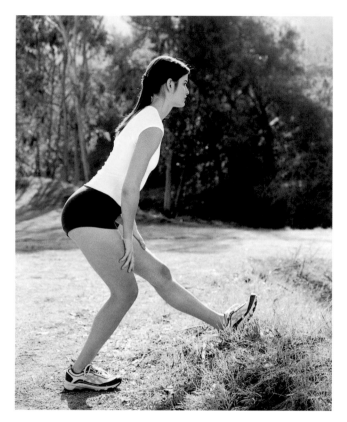

2. Hamstring stretch: Stand facing a curb or raised surface and place the heel of left foot on it, with left leg straight. Right leg is also straight, toes forward. Flex left foot toward you, squaring hips and shoulders to left leg. Sit back into right heel, bending right knee while bending torso forward at hips with back straight, until you feel a stretch at the back of left leg (as shown). Release and complete all reps, then switch legs.

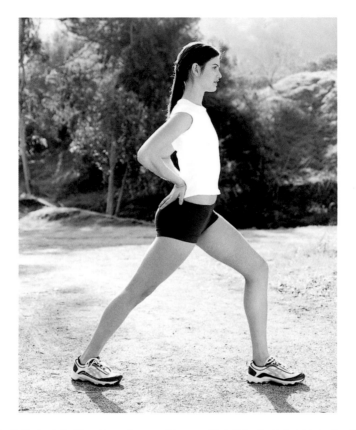

3. Calf stretch: Stand in a staggered lunge with left foot a full stride in front of right, feet hip-width apart, toes pointing straight ahead, and hands on hips. Bend left knee so that it's in line with left ankle; keep right leg straight and foot flat. Press hips gently forward, feeling stretch in right calf while keeping right heel on ground (as shown). Release, then repeat with right knee (back leg) bent to stretch underlying calf muscle. Complete all reps, then switch legs and repeat both stretches on other leg.

Ultimate Word

Don't be afraid to try a new cardio class. Just because you've mastered Spinning or kickboxing doesn't mean that you won't be nervous about trying the latest funky-dance class at your gym. "Sure, starting a new class is a little scary," says Gregory Florez, a spokesman for the American Council on Exercise. "But if you do your homework ahead of time, your first session won't be quite so nerve-wracking." Here are his suggestions:

- Peek in on a class during the most intense time. Don't look at the girl in the front row with the killer abs. Instead, steer your eyes toward the back of the room where the newer and less fit people usually gather. Are they keeping up?

- Grab someone on the way out of the class and ask her some questions: Does the instructor explain the movements? Does she modify them for different intensities?

- Remind yourself that everyone in the class was at your stage at some point, and that they're not in there to watch the new person who doesn't get all the steps.

- If all else fails, remember this: There's nothing embarrassing you can do that the instructor hasn't already seen!

The cardio workouts in this chapter don't take much time, but we know that sometimes your schedule makes even these sessions impossible to fit in. That's why we've devoted the next chapter to solving the time crunch and still looking great.

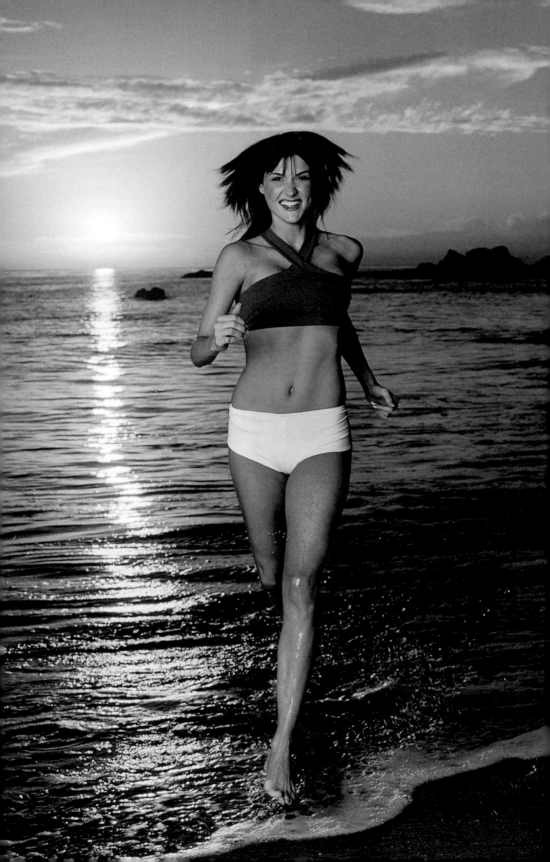

chapter 10

quick
do-anywhere
(no-excuses)
workouts

By now you know that you must stick to a regular exercise schedule to get and keep the Ultimate Body. You even *want* to exercise regularly, but sometimes it's tough to squeeze a full workout into your busy schedule.

This Chapter's To-Do List

In the following pages, you'll learn:

- How to eliminate excuses for not exercising

- Methods for working out with minimal equipment anywhere, anytime

- Ways to use multiple muscles at once to save time and blast fat

- 1-minute moves and 30-minute regimens to become stronger, more energized, and less stressed

"Hall of Lame" Excuses for Not Working Out

The quick, do-at-home workouts in this chapter eliminate many of the unsatisfactory excuses you may have for not going to the gym or out for a run—and we've heard them all. While some might be acceptable ("I'm in a full-body cast"), most of them don't hold water with us. Have you ever used any of these?

- "I can't go to the gym—I haven't shaved my legs in days."

- "The newspaper said there's a 20 percent chance it might rain."

- "But if I go for a walk before work I'll miss Matt Lauer on the *Today* show."

- "All my socks are in the wash."

- "I forgot the combination to my padlock."

- "My iPod/pedometer/heart-rate monitor is out of batteries."

- "I didn't pack my blow-dryer in my bag."

- "My cat/dog/parrot will miss me."

- "The holidays are coming—I'll wait until they're over."

- "I'll work out tomorrow."

If you answered yes to any of these bottom-of-the-barrel excuses, drop and give us 20 right now! And when you've finished, carry on and become familiar with our do-anywhere solutions.

One-Minute Workouts

It may sound too good to be true, but a number of published studies show that you can stay in shape and burn enough calories to maintain or lose weight by doing mini-workouts throughout the day. In fact, research has shown that short bouts of exercise—as few as three 10-minute sessions—are just as effective as 1 long workout, provided that the total cumulative time and intensity level are comparable, says exercise physiologist Glenn Gaesser, Ph.D., co-author of *The Spark: The Revolutionary New Plan to Get Fit and Lose Weight 10 Minutes at a Time.* That's where our 1-minute workouts come in.

Perform each of our 20 cardio or strength moves on its own, or mix and match several to create a longer regimen—one that's customized for you (such as our sample 10-, 20-, and 30-minute programs, which deliver on 3 of the most popular fitness goals). In terms of building aerobic fitness and stamina, Gaesser notes that it's necessary to work on increasing either the duration or intensity of your exercise. But in a pinch, these 1-minute moves can get you strong and energized, and make you more productive—without disrupting your day.

How it works: We've mapped out 10 strength moves and 10 cardio blasts, each of which takes about 1 minute to do. Aim to perform 1–5 of these every couple of hours, or all 10 all at once whenever you can squeeze them in. Ultimately, you should strive to get at least 30 minutes of physical activity on a day when you're getting your workout this way.

Warm-up: If you're only doing 1 move, no warm-up is necessary. If you plan to exercise for 10 minutes or longer, warm up with 1–3 minutes of light-cardio activity such as marching in place.

Cooldown: Even if you've only done 1 move, end each workout by stretching the muscle groups just worked, holding each stretch for 30 seconds without bouncing (stretch legs and back following your cardio moves).

One-Minute Strength Moves

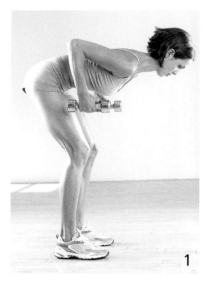

1. Bent-over row: Stand with a dumbbell in each hand, feet hip-width apart. Bend knees, flexing forward from hips until back is parallel to the floor, arms hanging in line with shoulders, and palms in. Bend elbows, pulling dumbbells in toward waist (as shown), then straighten arms. Do 4 reps, then use hamstrings to stand up. Repeat for 1 minute total.

Weight: 5- to 10-pound dumbbells. Strengthens back, rear shoulders, biceps, and hamstrings.

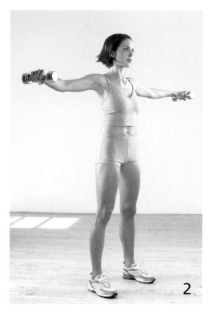

2. Five-time raise: Stand with a dumbbell in each hand, feet hip-width apart, arms hanging by sides, and palms in. Without rocking, lift arms out to sides and up to shoulder height (as shown), then lower. Do 5 reps, moving arms closer to midline of body with each lift (by rep 5, arms should raise directly in front of body at shoulder height). Repeat entire sequence for 1 minute total.

Weight: 3- to 5-pound dumbbells. Strengthens shoulders.

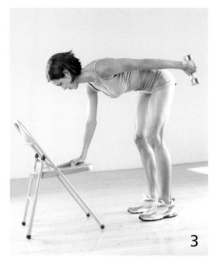

3. Kickback: Holding a dumbbell in your left hand, stand facing a chair. Bend forward from hips with knees slightly bent and place right hand on seat. Bend left elbow at waist to bring upper arm alongside torso, knuckles pointing down. Keeping elbow at waist, straighten left arm behind you (as shown). Repeat for 30 seconds (about 8–12 reps), then switch arms and repeat.

   Weight: 3- to 6-pound dumbbells. Strengthens triceps.

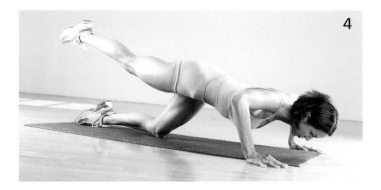

4. Push-up with alternating leg lift: Kneel on all fours with knees behind hips, hands just wider than shoulders, and abs contracted. Bend elbows and lower chest toward floor; simultaneously extend one leg up and behind to hip height (as shown). Straighten arms and lower knee to starting position. Repeat, alternating legs, for 1 minute total.

   Strengthens chest, triceps, buttocks, and hamstrings.

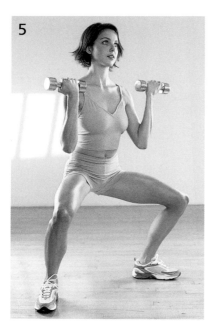

5. Plié with rotated biceps curl: With a dumbbell in each hand, stand with feet slightly more than hip-width apart, knees and toes turned out comfortably, arms hanging by sides, and palms in. Bend both knees and lowering hips without changing pelvis position. Simultaneously bend elbows, rotating dumbbell to face shoulder at top of move (as shown). Repeat for 1 minute total.

Weight: 5- to 8-pound dumbbells. Strengthens quadriceps, hamstrings, buttocks, adductors, and biceps.

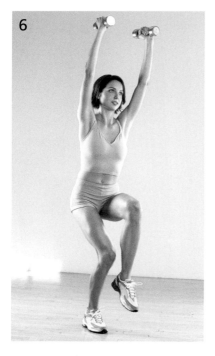

6. One-legged squat with overhead press: Hold a dumbbell in each hand, elbows bent close to sides with dumbbells at shoulder level, and palms in. Raise left leg, with left knee bent slightly and toes pointing down. Bend right knee into a squat, sitting back toward heel; simultaneously press weight up overhead (as shown). Straighten standing leg and lower weights. Repeat for 30 seconds (about 12–15 reps), then switch legs and repeat.

Weight: 5- to 8-pound dumbbells. Strengthens buttocks, hamstrings, quadriceps, calves, shoulders, and biceps.

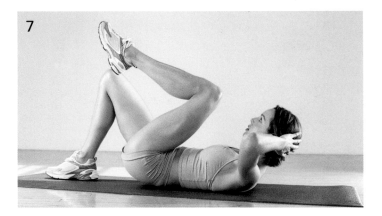

7. One-legged double crunch: Lie faceup with fingertips behind head, left knee in line with hips, calf raised and parallel to the floor, right foot on the floor, and knee bent. Contract abs, lifting upper torso until shoulder blades clear the floor, simultaneously lifting hips off the floor and bringing knee to chest. Hold position, tightening abs even further (as shown), then lower to starting position. Repeat for 30 seconds total, then switch legs.

Strengthens abdominals.

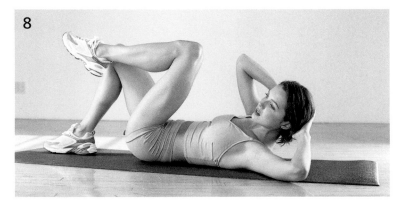

8. Alternating knee twist: Lie faceup with fingertips behind head, feet flat on the floor, and knees bent. Contract abs, lifting and bringing left knee in toward chest while rotating right shoulder toward left knee and keeping elbows open (as shown). Lower foot to the floor, then repeat with right knee and left shoulder. Alternate sides for 1 minute total.

Strengthens abdominals, especially obliques.

quick do-anywhere workouts

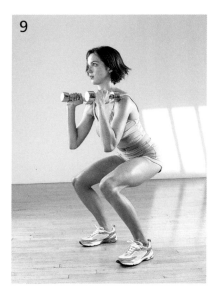

9. Squat with knee lift: Stand with feet hip-width apart and hands on hips (for a greater challenge, hold a dumbbell in each hand at shoulder height, palms in). With body weight toward heels, bend knees, lowering hips into a squat (as shown). Straighten legs and lift one knee up to hip height. Repeat, alternating knees, for 1 minute total.

Weight: 5- to 8-pound dumbbells.

Strengthens quadriceps, hamstrings, and buttocks.

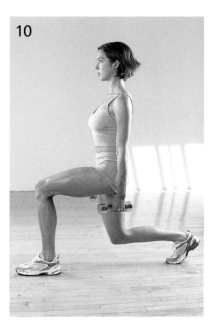

10. Rear lunge: Stand with feet hip-width apart and hands on hips (for a greater challenge, hold a dumbbell in each hand). Step backward with right foot, bending knees so that front knee aligns with ankle and back knee points down (as shown). Push off back foot to return to starting position. Repeat, alternating legs, for 1 minute total.

Weight: 5- to 8-pound dumbbells.

Strengthens quadriceps, hamstrings, buttocks, and calves.

One-Minute Cardio Moves

Repeat any of the following exercises for one minute total. (You can find some additional ideas in our Five-Minute-Workout Cardio Moves on page 246.)

1. Jumping jack: Stand with feet together, then jump, separating legs and raising arms overhead. Land with feet hip-width apart, then jump feet back together and lower arms.

2. Stair running: Run up a flight of stairs while pumping your arms, then walk down. Vary by taking two stairs at a time.

3. Jumping rope: Do a basic boxer's shuffle or two-footed jump. Stay on balls of feet, not jumping too high off the ground, keeping elbows by your sides.

4. Squat jump:* Stand with feet hip-width apart. Bend knees and lower hips into a squat. Jump in air and straighten legs, lifting arms upward. Land softly, lowering arms.

5. Split jump:* Stand in a split stance (one foot a long stride in front of the other), then bend knees and jump, switching legs to land and pumping arms in opposition to legs. Alternate legs.

6. Step-up:* Step up on a curb, stair, or sturdy bench with one foot, then the other; then step down one foot at a time. Repeat.

7. Alternating knee lift: Standing tall, bring one knee toward chest without collapsing rib cage; twist opposite elbow toward knee. Alternate sides.

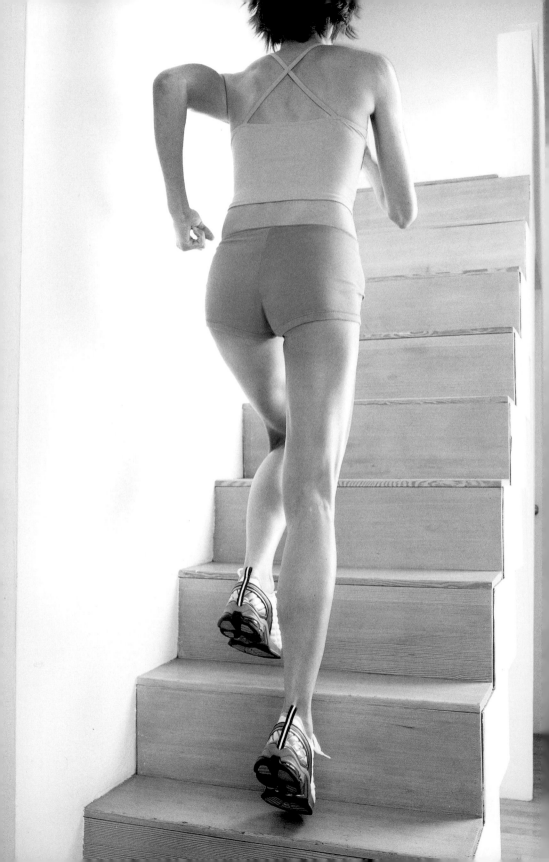

8. Hamstring curl:* Standing tall, step sideways with right foot, bringing left heel toward buttocks; pull elbows in to sides. Alternate sides.

9. Jog in place: Jog in place, lifting knees up and swinging arms naturally in opposition. Land softly, rolling from ball of foot to heel.

10. Side-to-side leap:* Place any long, thin object (such as a broom) on floor. Leap sideways over object, landing with feet together.

* Use these moves in our 10-Minute Butt-Blaster Workout.

Customized Workouts

This program has all the tools you need to build your own workout. Here are three examples to get you going—each one targets top exercise goals.

Workout 1: 10-Minute Butt Blaster

Guidelines: For a quick, tush-toning session, alternate cardio and strength moves that work your rear end. Warm up by doing one minute of light cardio activity. Do one butt-blasting cardio move (see starred cardio moves in the previous section) followed by one lower-body (or upper/lower-body combo) strength move; repeat this superset 5 times, varying the exercises each time. End your workout with 30-second stretches for all of your major muscle groups, with an emphasis on those for the lower body.

10 Minute Butt Blaster
Sample Workout:

Cardio:	Side-to-side leap
Strength:	Plié with rotated-biceps curl
Cardio:	Hamstring curl
Strength:	Rear lunge
Cardio:	Squat jump
Strength:	Squat with knee lift
Cardio:	Step-up
Strength:	Push-up with alternating-leg lift
Cardio:	Split jump
Strength:	One-legged squat with overhead press

Workout 2: 20-Minute Metabolism Booster

Guidelines: Boost your heart rate and blast calories by doing 5 cardio/strength circuits that work both your upper and lower body. Warm up by doing 2–3 minutes of light cardio activity. Then complete a circuit consisting of any three cardio moves, followed by 1 upper/lower-body combo strength move. Perform a total of 5 circuits. Do all 3 of the upper/lower-body-combo strength moves at least once. End your workout with 30-second stretches for all of your major muscle groups.

Sample workout:

Circuit 1:	Any 3 cardio moves, push-up with alternating-leg lift
Circuit 2:	Any 3 cardio moves, plié with rotated-biceps curl
Circuit 3:	Any 3 cardio moves, one-legged squat with overhead press
Circuit 4:	Any 3 cardio moves, push-up with alternating-leg lift
Circuit 5:	Any 3 cardio moves, plié with rotated-biceps curl

Workout 3: 30-Minute Total-Body Sculptor

Guidelines: For maximum definition and toning of your entire body, perform ten 3-minute cardio/strength circuits. Warm up by doing 2–3 minutes of light-cardio activity. Then complete a circuit consisting of any 2 cardio moves followed by 1 strength move. Do 10 circuits total, varying your exercises each time. Be sure to include all 10 strength exercises that we've prescribed in every workout. Occasionally change the order of your moves to add variety and bust boredom. End with 30-second stretches for all of your major muscle groups.

Sample workout:

Circuit 1: Any 2 cardio moves, plié with rotated biceps curl

Circuit 2: Any 2 cardio moves, rear lunge

Circuit 3: Any 2 cardio moves, one-legged squat with overhead press

Circuit 4: Any 2 cardio moves, bent-over row

Circuit 5: Any 2 cardio moves, squat with knee lift

Circuit 6: Any 2 cardio moves, five-time raise

Circuit 7: Any 2 cardio moves, push-up with alternating leg lift

Circuit 8: Any 2 cardio moves, kickback

Circuit 9: Any 2 cardio moves, one-legged double crunch

Circuit 10: Any 2 cardio moves, alternating knee twist

Five-Minute Workouts

In this exclusive program created by Mindy Mylrea, an American Council on Exercise–certified trainer based in Santa Cruz, California, you can order up a better body as simply as you would a fast-food meal (but with much healthier results!). Perhaps you'll be tempted by one of our 5-minute cardio or strength choices—or our 5-minute exercise combo for a leaner body. Or maybe you'll want to supersize by stringing together several 5-minute circuits for an even higher calorie burn and maximum definition. The choice is yours.

How it works: We've given you 5 strength moves and 10 cardio workouts. Put together any 5 whenever you have time to spare throughout your day, or combine enough moves to make a longer program. (See our sample workouts—including 3 options of only 5 minutes each and a 30-minute circuit program.) Just don't exceed 45 minutes at a time.

Warm-up: Before doing any of the 5-minute programs, perform 1 of the cardio moves at a lower intensity for 1 minute. If you plan on exercising for 10 minutes or more, warm up with 2–3 minutes of the light-cardio activity of your choice.

Cooldown: After your strength and/or cardio workout, stretch all of the major muscle groups that you just worked, holding each stretch for 30 seconds without bouncing (stretch legs and back following your cardio moves).

Misstep:

Letting one skipped workout turn into missing a week—and then several months—of exercise. A lapse becomes a habit when you forget the original reason that you missed a workout, and instead begin to focus on your guilt and the fear that you might miss even more. Transform those negative feelings into positive actions.

The first step is to think of guilt as an alarm clock that alerts you to the fact that you're not taking care of yourself. Then instead of focusing on the guilt, determine what caused your lapse and work to solve it (Are you too busy? Bored with your routine? Upset about something else?). Next comes what can be the hardest part: Be nice to yourself. That way, your feelings will help guide you toward your goal instead of pushing you away from it. The more you let negative self-talk into your life, the harder it is to get back on track. Instead, listen more closely to your needs.

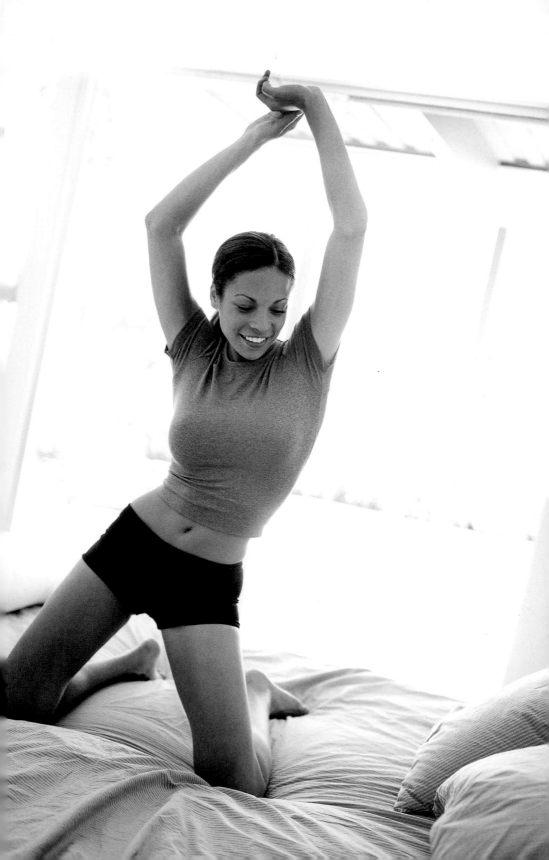

Strength Moves

Repeat each of the 5 moves as many times as you can for one minute, for a total of 5 minutes. For lunges, repeat for 30 seconds on each side.

Note: Be careful of the surface you do these moves on. One that's too slippery can cause you to slide out of control. Practice getting the feel of the paper plate under your feet before doing the exercises.

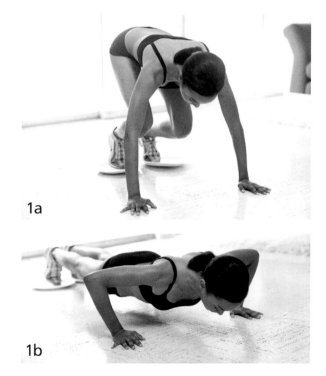

1a

1b

1. Push-up/pull-in: Kneeling with toes curled under, and a paper plate under the ball of each foot, walk hands forward until body is a straight line from head to heels, with knees lifted, abs contracted, and arms straight. Bend elbows, lowering entire body toward the floor and aligning elbows with shoulders (a). Press back up to starting position, then pull knees in toward chest by sliding feet on paper plates (b). Straighten legs and repeat.

Strengthens chest, front shoulders, triceps, quadriceps, hamstrings, buttocks, and abdominals.

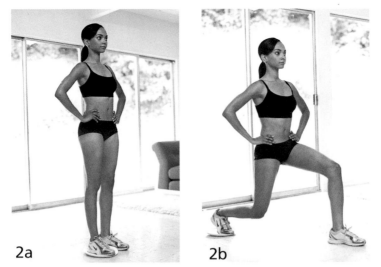

2a   2b

2. Plate lunge: Stand with feet hip-width apart, a paper plate under right foot, and hands on hips (a). Slide right foot back, bending both knees so that left knee aligns with left ankle, and right knee approaches the floor with heel lifted (b). Pull right foot back in, straightening legs to starting position. Repeat for 30 seconds, then switch legs.

For variety, slide right foot out to lunge to the right side, with right knee bent and aligning with right ankle, left leg straight.

Strengthens quadriceps, hamstrings, buttocks, calves, upper hips, and inner thighs.

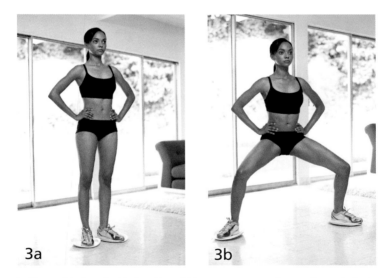

3a   3b

3. Plate plié: Stand with feet hip-width apart, a paper plate under each foot, hands on hips, and legs rotated out comfortably from hips. Contract abs and keep spine in a neutral position (a). Bend knees, sliding plates apart as wide as possible while keeping torso erect, tailbone pointing down, and knees aligned over feet (b). Using inner thighs, pull legs back together and repeat.

Strengthens quadriceps, inner thighs, hamstrings, and buttocks.

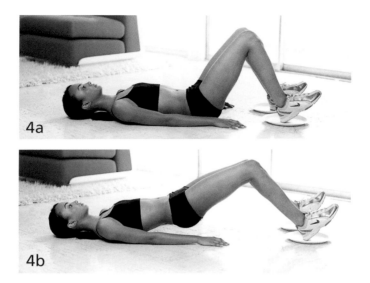

4. Plate bridge: Lie faceup with knees bent, a paper plate under each heel, toes lifted, and arms relaxed by your sides. Contract abs, bringing spine to a neutral position (a). Lift hips, sliding heels out only to the point that you can keep hips lifted and can slide heels back to starting position without arching back or dropping hips; keep toes lifted throughout (b). Pull heels toward you and lower hips to the floor; repeat.
Strengthens hamstrings, buttocks, abdominals, and spine extensors.

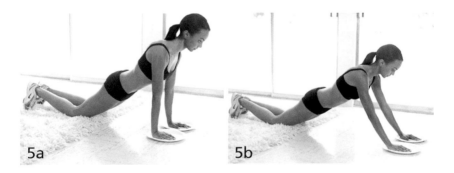

5. Plate-ab slide: Kneel on the floor, hips aligned over knees, each hand on a paper plate, wrists aligned under shoulders, and arms straight. Drop hips forward so that your body forms a straight line from shoulders to knees (a). Adjust hands forward, if necessary. Keeping arms straight, slide hands forward as far as possible while maintaining a straight torso (b). Slide plates back in, returning to starting position.
Strengthens abdominals, spine extensors, chest, and front shoulders.

Q. When my period comes, I'm just too tired to work, let alone exercise. Why does this happen?

A. "The exact reasons for changes in energy level with menses are not known," says Melissa Gilliam, M.D., M.P.H., assistant professor of obstetrics and gynecology at the University of Illinois at Chicago. If your symptoms start after day 14 of your cycle, it's likely they're due to PMS. "Low energy is definitely recognized as a PMS symptom, but it's not one of the more common ones," she says.

Recording your energy level throughout your menstrual cycle will help your doctor determine the cause of your problem. "Anemia and depression should be ruled out. Sometimes people ascribe low energy to their menstrual cycle when, in fact, they're not related," Gilliam cautions.

If your low energy is a symptom of PMS, try getting more exercise, even though you currently feel too tired to work out. "It's a little counterintuitive," she says, "but if you're active, you just feel better and have more energy, and you tend not to sink so low during PMS."

Cardio Moves

Repeat each move as many times as you can, at as high an intensity as you're able to maintain for 1 minute (this may vary by move). String together 5 moves for a 5-minute cardio blast. (For additional ideas, see One-Minute Workout Cardio Moves, page 235.)

1. Squat and kick: Step sideways with right foot so that feet are slightly more than hip-width apart, and squat. Straighten legs, bringing right foot back in, and immediately kick out to left side with left foot, then return to standing position. Repeat 4–8 times; switch sides. Continue to alternate sides.

2. Jumping jack/lunge combo: Alternate 1 jumping jack with 1 jump lunge (jump 1 foot forward and 1 back in a split stance, then jump feet back together). Repeat, alternating lunging leg with each combo.

3. Jump over the lines: Place 2 pieces of masking tape (or other markers) parallel to each other on the floor, about 3 feet apart. Standing between the markers, leap sideways to the left and land with both feet together outside of left marker. Leap back to center and repeat to right side of the marker, increasing speed or height of jump as you go.

4. Skate and foot tap: Hop on to left foot and bend right leg, lifting and crossing right foot behind left leg and tapping foot with left hand; repeat on opposite side and keep alternating until you've completed 8 hops. Then bring right knee to chest and tap right heel with right hand; repeat on opposite side, alternating until you've completed 8 taps. Continue, reducing reps to 4, then 2, then 1 of each or until you've completed 1 minute.

5. Stair run or step-up: Run up a flight of stairs while pumping your arms, then walk down. Vary by taking 2 stairs at a time. If you don't have access to stairs, step up and down on a bench or curb, alternating legs.

6. Shuffle/carioca: Stand at one side of a room or large area, your left side facing in toward the room. Shuffle sideways quickly to the opposite side of the room. Going back, "carioca," stepping out to side with right foot, cross left foot in front, step out to side again with right foot, cross left foot behind right, twisting hips in the direction you're moving. Continue until you reach the opposite side of the room. Repeat shuffle, then carioca, starting with left foot this time.

7. Run/backpedal: Stand at one side of a room or large area. Run forward to the opposite side, then return to the starting point by running backward.

8. Squat jump 1+2: Stand with feet hip-width apart. Bend knees and lower hips to a quarter-squat, then jump up while straightening legs and lifting arms upward. Land softly, lowering hips to a deeper squat, thighs as parallel to the floor as possible; repeat entire combo.

9. Long jump: Stand 5–10 feet behind a piece of tape. Run up to it and then jump past it with both feet or leap past it with one foot (landing on both feet or just one if you're up to the challenge). Mark your landing. Walk back to the starting point and repeat, each time trying to outdo previous distance.

10. Roll the dice: Jog in place and toss 2 dice. Add the numbers and multiply the total by 2, then perform that many jumping jacks. Repeat. Alternatively, do this with any of your favorite moves, such as squat and kick or squat jump 1+2.

Slip Sliding Away

If you like this workout but don't want to keep an unlimited supply of paper plates in the house, you might want to invest in a set of Gliding Discs. They're lightweight, Frisbee-like discs that let you slide fluidly through strength and core exercises with a wide range of motion, even on carpet. When you buy them, you'll also get a DVD or VHS tape with further exercises. Find them at **http:// glidingdiscs.com.**

Customized Workouts

Workout 1: Tighter Buns

Guidelines: For toning your lower body, perform either a "strength sandwich" (1 cardio move, then 3 lower-body-strength moves, followed by 1 cardio move), or a "cardio sandwich" (1 lower-body-strength move, then 3 cardio moves, followed by 1 strength move).

Sample "strength sandwich" workouts:
1. Skate and foot tap, plate plié, plate bridge, plate-ab slide, skate and foot tap
2. Stair run or step-up, plate lunge, plate plié, plate lunge, stair run or step-up

Sample "cardio sandwich" workouts:

1. Plate bridge, jumping jack/lunge combo,
    jump over the lines, skate and foot tap, plate plié
2. Plate lunge, stair run or step-up, shuffle/carioca,
    squat jump 1+2, plate bridge

Workout 2: Extra Lean

Guidelines: To get maximum calorie burn, do a cardio/strength combo consisting of any 2 cardio moves, then 1 strength move, followed by 2 cardio moves.

Sample workouts:

1. Squat and kick, jump over the lines,
    plate lunge, jumping jack/lunge combo, roll the dice,
2. Shuffle/carioca, squat jump 1+2, plate lunge,
    skate and foot tap, shuffle/carioca.

Workout 3: Supersize Your Exercise

Guidelines: You'll get a total-body tone-up and maximum fat blast by increasing your workout to 30 minutes. Perform 6 circuits (each lasting 5 minutes), combining either 3 cardio and 2 strength moves, or 3 strength and 2 cardio moves. Recover as needed after each circuit with a light jog or walk for 30–90 seconds. Progress by decreasing the rest time between circuits.

Sample workouts:

Perform 1 of these sample circuits 6 times, doing each
of them in the order listed, or mix and match any of
the strength and cardio moves to create your own program.

Circuit 1:   Jump over the lines, plate bridge, stair run or step-up, plate lunge, run/backpedal

Circuit 2:   Skate and foot tap, push-up/pull-in, jump over the lines, plate-ab slide, run/backpedal

Circuit 3:   Squat and kick, plate plié, jumping jack/lunge combo, push-up/pull-in, long jump

Circuit 4:   Plate plié, squat jump 1+2, plate bridge, long jump, plate-ab slide

Circuit 5:   Plate lunge, squat and kick, push-up/pull-in, roll the dice, plate plié

Her Ultimate Turning Point

Jessica Norwick of Illinois broke down and cried when she saw herself in family photographs weighing 165 pounds. Then she began doing some form of exercise five times a week. "I felt too self-conscious to go to the gym," she says, "so I worked out at home on a treadmill." After a couple of workouts, she felt good that she was doing something positive for her health. She also developed healthy eating habits and lost 30 pounds over the next 4 months—but then she hit a plateau and turned to junk food out of frustration. After regaining 7 pounds, she got back on the program, and eventually reached her goal weight of 125 pounds.

Her Best Tip: Change your workout routine every few weeks—for Jessica, it's every 6–8 weeks—so that your body is always challenged.

Ten-Minute Workout

Compound moves are the key to this short-circuit strength-training workout. The program will tone your entire body with 6 incredible moves designed by Annette Lang, a Reebok University Master Trainer in New York City. "You're not just sitting on some machine isolating your muscles," she says. "Your entire body is involved in each move, so you're getting a lot more bang for your buck." You'll be working multiple muscle groups at once—up to 8 in a single exercise—while putting your balance and coordination to the test.

How it works: Do this program 2–4 times a week, with at least 1 day of rest between workouts. Perform 1 set of each exercise in the order listed, resting only long enough to set up for the next exercise; this equals 1 circuit. If you use 5- to 8-pound weights, do 15–20 reps for each exercise. If you use 8- to 10-pound weights, do 12–15 reps. To progress, lift heavier weights or add more circuits.

Warm-up: Begin with 5 minutes of light walking or stair climbing. Then do squats without weights, raising your arms over your head as you stand back up. As you squat, alternate the direction of your arms so that your hands reach directly overhead, then over your right shoulder, and then over your left. Do 10–15 reps with hands reaching in each direction.

Cooldown: Finish your workout by stretching all of your major muscle groups, holding each stretch for 20–30 seconds without bouncing, and repeating each stretch 2 or 3 times.

The Moves

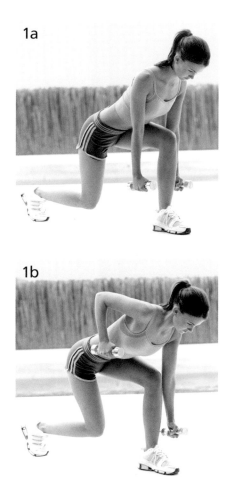

1a

1b

1. Diagonal lunge with row: Standing with feet hip-width apart, hold a dumbbell in each hand with arms by sides. Contract abs so that spine is in a neutral position. Take a slightly diagonal step forward to place left foot at "11 o'clock," then bend knees so that left knee aligns with left ankle and right knee approaches the ground with heel lifted. At the same time, bend forward from hips with lower back flat and reach dumbbells toward left foot, palms facing in (a). Maintaining diagonal lunge, bend right elbow back toward waist in a rowing motion (b). Straighten right arm, then push back to starting position and repeat entire move on opposite side, lunging with right foot at "1 o'clock." Continue alternating to complete all reps on each side.

Strengthens quadriceps, hamstrings, buttocks, calves, spine extensors, shoulders, and biceps.

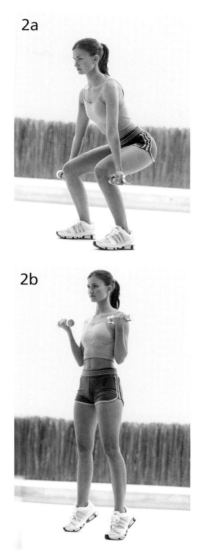

2a

2b

2. Squat combo: Standing with feet hip-width apart, hold a dumbbell in each hand with arms by sides, elbows in line with shoulders, and palms facing forward. Contract abs so that tailbone points to the floor and spine is in a neutral position. With body weight toward heels, bend knees to lower hips into a squat until thighs are almost parallel to the ground (a). Straighten legs to full standing position, then lift onto balls of feet in a calf raise; at the same time, bend elbows, curling dumbbells in toward shoulders (b). Straighten arms and lower heels, then repeat entire combo.
Strengthens quadriceps, hamstrings, buttocks, calves, and biceps.

3a

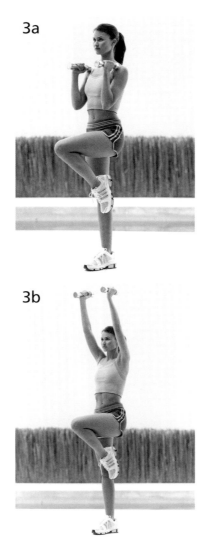

3b

3. One-legged overhead press: Standing with feet hip-width apart, hold a dumbbell in each hand with elbows bent close to torso, heads of dumbbells at shoulder height, and palms facing in. Contract abs so that spine is in a neutral position, then balance and lift one foot off the ground a few inches with knee slightly bent (for more of a challenge, bend knee to hip height, as shown) (a). Maintain one-legged position and straighten arms overhead (b). Lower arms and repeat overhead press for half of the reps, then switch legs for the other half. For the ultimate challenge, bend supporting knee into a quarter-squat as arms lift overhead, straightening leg as arms lower.

Strengthens upper back, front and middle shoulders, buttocks, hamstrings, and quadriceps; abdominals and spine extensors act as stabilizers.

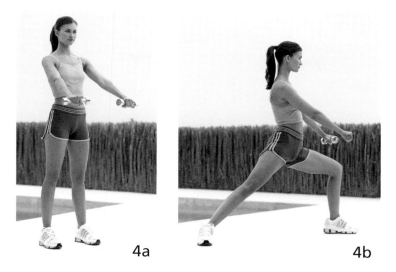

4a 4b

4. Lateral lunge with rotation: Standing with feet about 6 inches apart, hold a dumbbell in each hand with arms extended in front of body at lower-rib-cage height, palms down. Contract abs so that spine is in a neutral position (a). Step sideways with left foot, bend knee and turn toe out slightly, keeping knee in line with toes and right leg straight. As you lunge, rotate torso, bringing straight arms toward the lunging leg and keeping hips square (b). Rotate arms back to center while stepping feet together. Complete all reps, then switch sides to do all reps on opposite leg.

Strengthens quadriceps, hamstrings, buttocks, upper hips, inner thighs, front shoulders, upper chest, and abdominals.

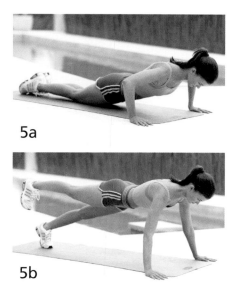

5a

5b

5. Push-up one-legged plank: Kneel on the ground with arms straight and slightly more than shoulder-width apart. Press hips forward, contracting abs until body forms a line from shoulders to knees; then bend elbows out to sides, lowering torso toward the ground (a). Press up, straightening arms and lifting knees, and balance on balls of feet; then lift one leg up to hip height (b). Lower leg, then bend knees onto ground and repeat, alternating leg lifts until you've completed all reps on each side.

Strengthens chest, front shoulders, triceps, and buttocks; abdominals and spine extensors as stabilizers.

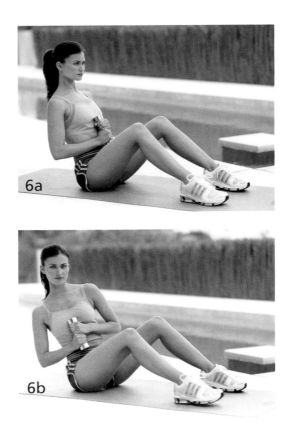

6. Seated rotated twist: Sit on the ground with knees bent and feet flat; or if possible, lift feet, bend knees in line with hips, and keep calves parallel to ground. Hold a dumbbell vertically with both hands in front of rib cage, keeping elbows bent and close to sides. Contract abs to maintain upright posture (a). Slowly rotate torso to one side, aiming lower part of dumbbell toward hip (b), then rotate to opposite side and continue to alternate until you've completed all reps on each side.

Strengthens abdominals and spine extensors.

30-Minute Workout

Even when you have the time to devote to your workout, there's nothing wrong with getting it done quickly, as long as you use those minutes effectively. *Shape* teamed up with kinesiologists Stuart Rugg, Ph.D., and Bill Whiting, Ph.D., to find the best exercises that you could possibly do to shape specific body parts. Using an electromyograph (EMG) machine, our science gurus recorded activity in different muscles as a test subject performed an assortment of popular moves.

Over a period of several months, we analyzed more than 125 exercises to come up with a master list of all-time "best-tested moves." The 8 we've selected here give you a supereffective total-body workout in 30 minutes. Since the program is designed as a circuit (that is, you go from one exercise to the next without resting), you'll blow through it faster, and you'll also get your heart rate up for an increased calorie burn.

Guidelines: Do this workout 3–4 times per week, taking a day off between each session. Perform 1 set (10–15 reps) of each exercise in the order listed without resting between sets, then complete the circuit a second time. For Moves 1–6 use 5- to 10-pound dumbbells. If you want to use more weight, you can cut back on reps, but don't drop below 8 reps per exercise. If you're an experienced lifter, or to advance, perform 3 circuits.

Mega-calorie-burning option: Add 2–3 minutes of cardio after every other move. For example, after you finish Moves 1 and 2, do 2–3 minutes of jogging in place, jumping rope, jumping jacks, or any other heart-pumping activity that you enjoy. Review the cardio moves in our One-Minute Workout (page 229) and Five-Minute Workout (page 240) for other ideas.

Warm-up: Do 5 minutes of any low-intensity cardio, such as brisk walking, marching in place, or step-ups.

Cooldown: End by stretching all of the major muscles worked, holding each stretch for 20–30 seconds without bouncing.

The Moves

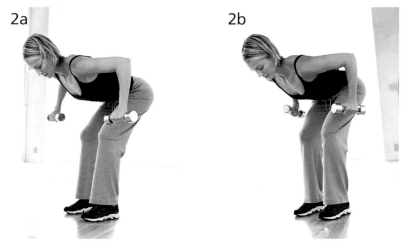

1. Front/rear lunge: Standing with feet hip-width apart, hold a dumbbell in each hand, arms by sides, and palms in. Take a large step forward with right foot, bending knees so that right knee aligns with right ankle and left knee approaches floor (a). Push back to starting point, then immediately lunge backward with right leg (b). Alternate front and rear lunges for all reps, then switch legs and repeat.

Strengthens quadriceps, hamstrings, buttocks, and calves.

2. Bent-over dumbbell row combo: Stand holding dumbbells with feet hip-width apart. Bend knees, then bend forward from hips until back is about parallel to the floor with arms hanging down and palms facing rear. Squeeze shoulder blades, then bend elbows up and out to shoulder height (a). Straighten arms to starting position, turn palms in, and pull elbows back toward waist, keeping torso still (b). Complete all reps.

Strengthens major muscles of the upper and middle back, middle and rear shoulders.

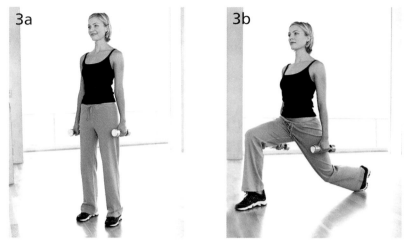

3. Walking lunge: Stand with feet hip-width apart and legs straight, holding dumbbells with arms by sides and palms in (a). Keeping abs contracted and chest lifted, take a large step forward with right foot, bending knees so that right knee aligns with ankle and left knee points down (b). Straighten legs and take a big step forward with left foot into another lunge. Continue alternating for all reps.

Strengthens quadriceps, upper hip, inner thighs, calves, hamstrings (somewhat), and buttocks.

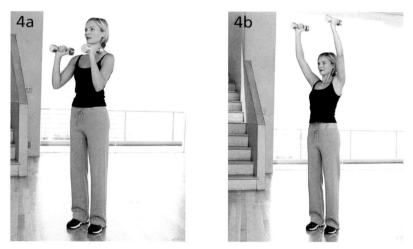

4. Overhead dumbbell press: Stand holding dumbbells with feet hip-width apart, legs straight, elbows bent at shoulder height, forearms parallel, and palms in. Contract abs and relax shoulders, keeping body upright (a). Using back and shoulder muscles, press arms upward; keep wrists straight and don't lock elbows (b). Lower to starting position; complete all reps.

Strengthens major muscles of the upper and middle back, shoulders, and biceps (somewhat).

quick do-anywhere workouts

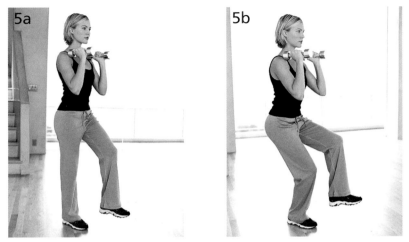

5. One-legged squat: Stand with feet hip-width apart and dumbbells on shoulders (beginners use no weight and place hands on hips). Lift left foot, using abdominals to stay balanced on right leg (a). Bend right knee and sit into as low a squat as possible (b). Contract buttocks and straighten right knee. Complete all reps, then switch legs and repeat.

Strengthens quadriceps, inner and outer thighs, buttocks, and hamstrings.

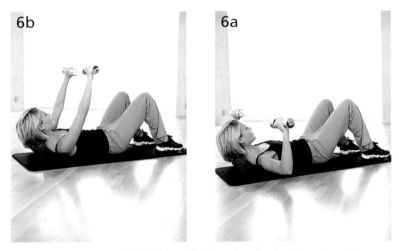

6. Chest press: Lie on back with a rolled towel under shoulders, knees bent, and feet flat. Grasping dumbbells, extend arms above chest with wrists straight and palms facing forward. Contract abs so that back is in contact with floor (a). Squeeze shoulder blades, then bend elbows out and down until they're in line with shoulders (b). Straighten arms, contracting chest muscles while pressing dumbbells up to starting position; complete all reps.

Strengthens chest, front shoulders, and triceps.

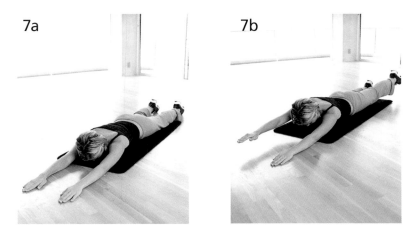

7. Prone alternating arm and leg raise: Lie facedown on floor with arms and legs extended. Contract abs to pull navel up off the floor and drop tailbone so that spine is in a neutral position (a). Maintaining abdominal contraction, lift right arm and left leg up off the floor (b). Lower, then repeat with opposite arm and leg. Continue alternating sides for all reps.

Strengthens back muscles (erector spinae), shoulders, and buttocks.

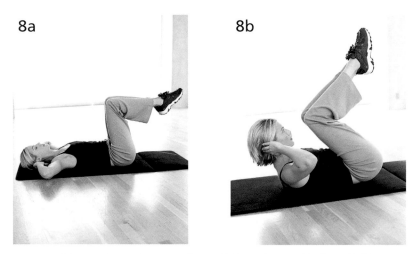

8. Double crunch: Lie faceup on floor with knees bent and in line with hips, calves parallel to the floor. Place fingertips behind head without clasping, keeping elbows open. Contract abs to pull navel in toward spine so that back is in contact with the floor (a). Use your abdominals to lift hips off the floor, simultaneously bringing knees toward chest and lifting head and shoulders up (b). Lower and complete all reps.

Strengthens abdominals.

Ultimate Word

Make sure that you get the most bang for your buck out of these quick workouts with these dos and don'ts.

Do . . .

- Vary the intensity of your cardio and elevate your heart rate enough.
- Choose workouts that are challenging enough and fatigue your target muscle.
- Take in fewer calories than you're burning.

Don't . . .

- Do the same workout routine every single time without mixing it up.
- Stick to only isolation exercises (instead of multimuscle moves).
- Overtrain your trouble zones to the exclusion of other important muscle groups.
- Work at too high an intensity, and/or not give your body enough time off between workouts.
- Quit when you plateau.

Many of the moves you've worked with so far can be done in the gym, and many are perfect for working out at home. In the next chapter, we're going to focus more closely on how to get the most benefits from the weight room at your health club—and the best ways to use it in achieving your Ultimate Body.

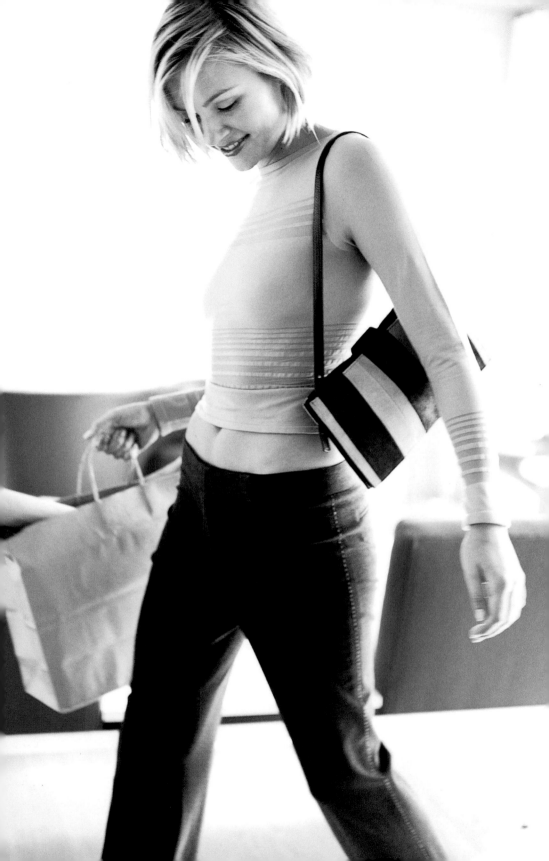

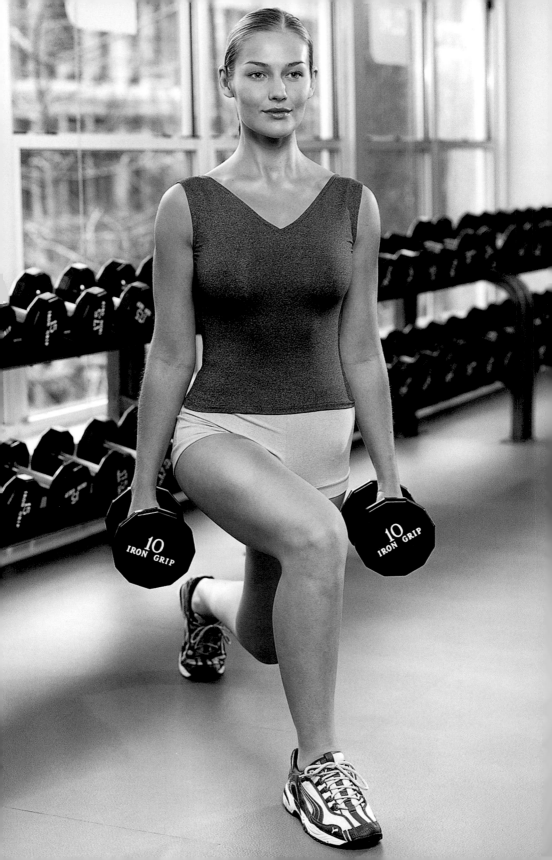

chapter 11

weight-room workouts

Undoubtedly, you can get a great workout at home with dumbbells and other equipment. But after a while, the same old sets and reps aren't going keep you on the road to your Ultimate Body. Going to the gym can help take your program to the next level by promoting greater muscle gain, jolting your metabolism, pushing you past a plateau, supercharging your motivation, and providing inspiration.

This Chapter's To-Do List

In the following pages, you'll learn:

- How to find a gym that's right for you
- Ways to lose weight with strength training
- The best methods for targeting your trouble zones
- Plateau-busting techniques
- The secrets to getting maximum results in the gym

Joining a Gym

Joining a gym can be a financial commitment, as well as an investment in your health and fitness. To ensure that you attend on a regular basis, you'll want to make sure that the club you belong to meets your needs and is a pleasant place that you'll look forward to going to. *Before you sign any long-term contracts, ask the following questions:*

1. Is it convenient to home or work? The easier it is to get to, the more likely you are to go.

2. Are sales staff and front-desk personnel helpful and friendly? Gyms can be intimidating to the uninitiated, and you want to feel welcome no matter what your level of fitness is.

3. Can you get a short-term trial membership to see if it suits you? Some places require lengthy commitments, and you want to be sure that you're making the right choice.

4. Is the equipment well maintained, and are the locker rooms clean and safe?

5. Do trainers and class instructors have training and certification from nationally recognized fitness agencies?

6. Do new members get instruction on how to use equipment?

7. Does it provide the cardio machines or classes you need (and like) to achieve your goals?

8. Is it crowded, with people standing around waiting to use the equipment when you most want to work out? Evenings are the busiest times for most health clubs; if that's when you plan to go, check it out then rather than during the day when it will most likely be relatively uncrowded.

9. Are babysitting and parking available if you need them?

10. Have you read the fine print in the contract?

If you answered yes to all of these questions, then it sounds like this gym is a good bet for you.

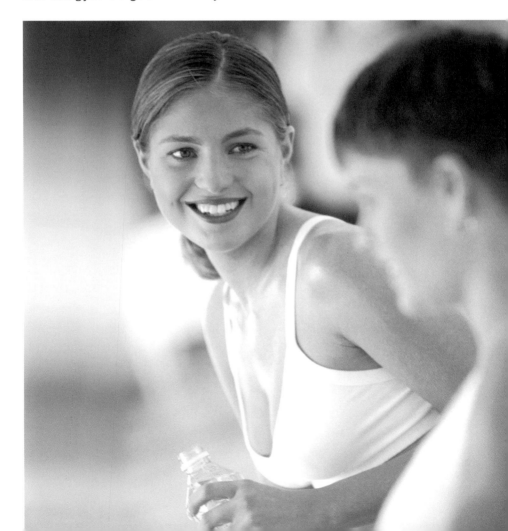

Q. What should I look for in a gym's contract?

A. It's important to know exactly what you're committing to when you sign the contract—and how you can cancel it if you end up unhappy. Don't be rushed. Take your time reading all of the paperwork—bring it home if you have to—and ask about anything that you don't understand.

"In a quality club, the rep is not going to be put off by showing you what's in the contract in detail," says Bill Howland, Jr., director of research at the International Health, Racquet, and Sportsclub Association in Boston. "If they don't have the willingness to go through it [with you], that should be a red flag."

Read the fine print. The "Financial Policy" section tells you what you pay; ask if any other charges (such as an additional fee for classes or monthly billing) are added to the cost. Un-less your membership is prepaid or the contract states that your monthly dues are frozen for life, most clubs reserve the right to increase rates as they see fit. And if there's anything extra (such as a free month) that the sales rep adds on as an incentive to get you to join, ask them to put it in writing.

Pay special attention to the "Cancellation" or "Termination" section. Make sure you're clear about how much notice you have to give if you wish to end your membership, and whether you have to submit that request in writing. Most clubs give you a three- to seven-day cooling-off period to change your mind right after you sign up and then require at least a 30-day written notice to cancel, but this varies from gym to gym. No federal law governs health-club contracts, but you should be able to cancel if you move more than 25 miles from the facility or an injury puts you out of commission.

If your gym won't honor the terms of its contract, and you can't get any resolution through the manager, contact your state attorney general's office. They can tell you whether there have been other complaints. Another option: File a complaint with the Federal Trade Commission (**ftc.gov** or 877-FTC-HELP). If you've followed your club's instructions, but they won't cancel your contract, and your monthly dues are automatically charged to your credit card, call your credit-card company to dispute the charges.

Goal-Oriented Workouts

You've probably tended to join a gym when you have a specific goal in mind: Perhaps you've wanted to lose weight, improve a particular body part, or reach a new level of fitness after you've stopped making progress in your home workouts. If you want to transform your physique, however, you need a customized program to get you there.

Andrea Bowman, a certified trainer based in Virginia Beach, Virginia, has designed an ultra-effective program for each of the three most common reasons that people join gyms: losing weight, targeting trouble zones, and busting a plateau. You'll start by learning 6 essential moves, and then you'll incorporate them into a plan custom-designed for what you want to achieve. We also alert you to the most common fitness faux pas associated with each goal, so you can avoid the mistakes that sabotage results.

The Essential Moves

Warm-up: Begin with 5–10 minutes of low-intensity exercise on any piece of cardio equipment.

Cooldown: End your workout with a static stretch for all of your major muscle groups, holding each stretch for about 30 seconds without bouncing.

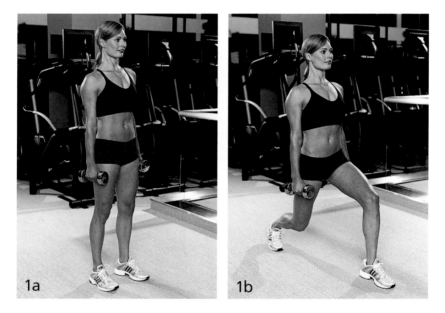

1a   1b

1. Front lunge: Stand with feet hip-width apart, holding a dumbbell in each hand with arms hanging at sides and palms in. Contract abs, bringing spine to a neutral position, and draw shoulder blades down and together (a). Take a large step forward with left foot, bending both knees so that left knee aligns with left ankle and right knee points toward floor with heel lifted (b). Push back to starting position with left foot, then complete all recommended reps on that side. Without resting, switch legs and repeat on opposite side to complete one set.

Weight: 5–20 pounds in each hand.

Strengthens quadriceps, hamstrings, buttocks, and calves.

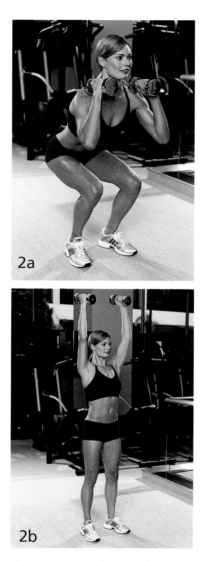

2. Squat with overhead press: Standing with feet hip-width apart, rest a dumbbell on each shoulder with elbows bent and palms in. Contract abs and draw shoulder blades down and together. Keeping body weight toward heels, lower hips until knees are bent at about 90 degrees (a). Return to standing position, then extend arms to press dumbbells directly overhead (b). Bend arms, returning dumbbells to starting position, and repeat combo.

Weight: 5–15 pounds in each hand.

Strengthens quadriceps, hamstrings, buttocks, upper back, and front and middle shoulders.

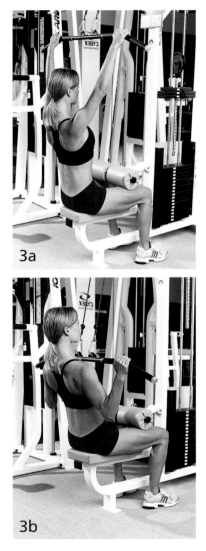

3a

3b

3. Lat pull-down: Attach a long bar to a lat-pull-down machine and adjust seat so that thighs are touching thigh pad when seated. Grasp bar with an overhand grip that's slightly wider than shoulder-width, then sit with feet flat on the floor, knees bent, and arms straight. Lean back slightly from hips so that bar is above chest (a). With abs contracted and shoulder blades drawn down and together, use back muscles to pull elbows down and in toward waist while lifting chest toward bar (b). Straighten arms to starting position and repeat.

Weight: 40–90 pounds.

Strengthens middle back and rear shoulders.

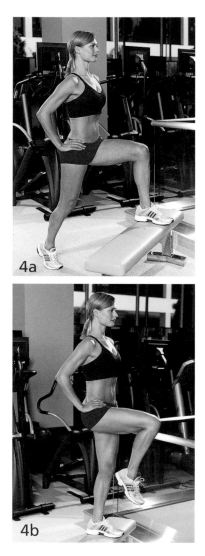

4. Step-up knee lift: Stand facing an 8- to 12-inch step or flat bench with hands on hips. Place left foot on top and in center of bench, knee bent and aligned with ankle, right leg straight, and heel lifted (a). With abs contracted and torso upright, bend right knee and push off right foot, using hip and thigh muscles to straighten both legs to lift up onto bench; bend right knee to hip height (b). Keep left foot on bench, lower right foot to floor, and complete reps; then repeat on opposite side to complete 1 set.

Strengthens quadriceps, hamstrings, buttocks, and calves.

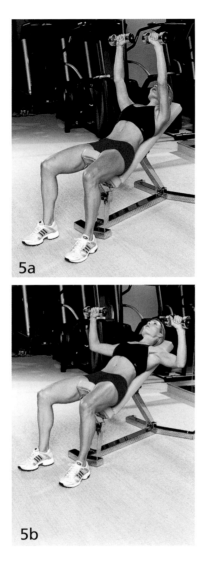

5a

5b

5. Incline dumbbell chest press: Adjust an incline bench to 30 degrees, then sit with back and hips against back pad, knees bent and in line with ankles. Hold a dumbbell in each hand, arms extended above midchest, palms facing forward, and wrists straight. Contract abs, bringing spine to a neutral position (a). Lower dumbbells out and down to sides until elbows are bent at 90 degrees and wrists align with elbows (b). Contract chest muscles to press weights back up to starting position and repeat.

Weight: 5–15 pounds in each hand.

Strengthens chest, front shoulders, and triceps.

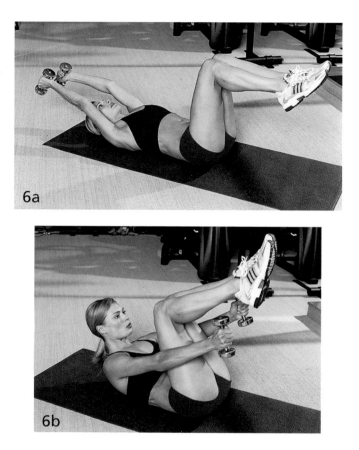

6. Double crunch: Lie faceup on the floor, knees bent in line with hips, and calves parallel to floor. Extend both arms behind head with palms in, contracting abs to bring spine to a neutral position (a). Lift arms, head, neck, and shoulder blades up off the floor, reaching arms toward ankles; at the same time, use abs to bring hips off floor (b). Lower and repeat.

Power Rx: Hold a 2- to 6-pound dumbbell in each hand.
Strengthens abdominals.

Goal 1: Lose Weight

Guidelines: This program is designed to boost your calorie burn for fast, effective weight loss. Besides sculpting your body, the strength-training exercises will help elevate your resting metabolism, which is the number of calories that you burn at rest. To maximize lean muscle mass, you'll lift heavy weights twice a week (but don't worry, you won't bulk up). Once a week, you'll do a strength circuit for an intense, fat-blasting workout.

With the strength moves, you'll work multiple muscle groups at once—a time-efficient way to train and strengthen your core, stabilizing muscles as a bonus. The cardio plan includes interval training (alternating spurts of high- and moderate-intensity exercise) to amp up your heart rate. Working at a high intensity will allow you to burn more calories both during the session and for several hours afterward.

Misstep:

Sabotaging your weight-loss success by:

- Doing the same cardio workout all the time.

- Not varying the intensity of your exercise or elevating your heart rate enough.

- Avoiding weight training or not using enough resistance.

- Only doing isolation exercises (instead of multimuscle moves).

- Taking in more calories then you're burning.

Strength: Follow the directions below, taking a day off between each weight-training workout.

Day 1: Do 2–3 sets (8–10 reps each) of all 6 Essential Moves (but do 12–15 reps of the step-up knee lifts with each leg without resting between sets). Where applicable, use enough resistance to fatigue your muscles by the final rep in each set; rest 30–60 seconds between sets.

Day 2: Do all of the exercises as a circuit: Perform 1 set of 12–15 reps using moderate weight for each, without resting between sets; this equals 1 circuit. Repeat for 2–3 circuits total. For an even bigger calorie burn, incorporate 2 minutes of any type of cardio after every other strength move.

Day 3: Repeat the workout from Day 1.

Cardio: Do 30–45 minutes of moderate-intensity, steady-state cardio 2–3 days a week. In addition, do 20–30 minutes of interval training (alternating 3–4 minutes at a moderate intensity with 2–3 minutes at a higher intensity) 2–3 days a week.

Goal 2: Target Your Trouble Zones

Guidelines: No matter what your trouble zone, this program can help improve it. The strength workout targets almost all of your major muscles for head-to-toe sculpting and symmetry. For maximum definition, you'll use a technique called a "superset" to intensify your workouts. Throughout the week, you'll also vary your resistance to stimulate more muscle fibers and enhance your results. The cardio plan incorporated interval training to incinerate calories and get rid of flab.

Superset 1: Front lunge, step-up knee lift, lat pull-down, double crunch

Superset 2: Squat with overhead press, incline dumbbell chest press, double crunch

Misstep:

Sabotaging your targeted workout by:

- Overtraining your trouble zone to the exclusion of other important muscle groups.

- Avoiding new exercises or not changing your routine.

- Doing workouts that aren't challenging enough, so your target muscles don't fatigue.

- Not burning enough calories to shed body fat.

Strength: Do the Essential Moves in a superset format as outlined above. Perform this workout 3 times a week, taking a day off between workouts. Do 1 heavy-lifting day and 2 moderate-lifting days each week. For each superset, do 1 set (8–10 reps on heavy days, 12–15 reps on moderate days) of each move back-to-back, without resting between sets. Then take a 30- to 40-second break, or up to 2 minutes if you need it. Do each superset 2–3 times before moving on. For variety, perform the exercises within the supersets in a different order each week. On all days, use enough resistance to fatigue your target muscles by the end of each set.

Cardio: Do 30–40 minutes of cardio a minimum of 4 days a week. At least once a week, ramp up your intensity by doing intervals (alternating 2 minutes at moderate intensity with 4 minutes at moderate to high intensity).

Goal 3: Break Through a Plateau

Guidelines: If you're no longer making progress in your fitness goals, chances are that your body has adapted to your routine. With this program, you'll stimulate your muscles and cardiovascular system in a variety of ways to push past the plateau and boost your fitness level. To shake up your strength workouts, you'll do a different number of reps and sets each time. Plus, you'll switch the order of your exercises every week. The cardio plan involves altering the intensity of your workouts and the activity you select—ideally, no 2 cardio workouts will be the same from week to week. To combat overtraining, be sure to take at least 1 day off a week.

Misstep:

Sabotaging your plateau-busting workout by:

- Doing the same workout routine every single time, and not mixing it up.

- Overtraining (working at too high an intensity and/or not taking enough time off between workouts).

- Quitting when progress stops.

Strength: Do the Essential Moves 3 times a week, taking a day off between workouts. Complete 1 heavy-, 1 moderate-, and 1 light-lifting day each week. On heavy days, do 2 sets of 6–8 reps. On moderate days, do 2–3 sets of 8–12 reps. On light days, do 3 sets of 12–15 reps. Always use enough resistance to fatigue your target muscles by the final rep. Rest 60–90 seconds between sets (or longer on heavy days).

Change the order of the exercises every week, as follows: For Week 1, do the Essential Moves in the order listed; reverse the order for Week 2; in the third week, do even numbers followed by odd numbers; and finish up in week 4 by doing odd numbers followed by even. Then return to the Week-1 instructions.

Cardio: Do 4–5 cardio workouts a week, varying your intensity as follows: Once a week, do 30–45 minutes of moderate, steady-state cardio; and 25–30 minutes of interval training (alternating 1 minute at a high intensity with 2–3 at a low intensity). Then 2–3 times a week, do 30–40 minutes of moderate cardio, slightly raising or lowering your intensity every few minutes. Try to do a different cardio activity or use a different machine each time.

Her Ultimate Turning Point

Jewel Heisig of Colorado made one attempt to lose weight and improve her health: She joined a gym. But at 250 pounds, she felt too self-conscious to go. Six months before her unused membership expired, Jewel's sister-in-law mentioned that she wanted to get in shape for a wedding. When she found out that Jewel's membership allowed her to bring a guest to the gym for free, she asked Jewel to take her.

The two women started their fitness program by walking on the treadmill. Within a month, Jewel was walking, biking, or stair climbing 4–5 times a week. As the weeks progressed, the pounds started to drop off, and Jewel felt more energetic. She added weight training and sensible eating to her program. As a result, she lost 110 pounds in a year.

"When I was overweight, being fit and healthy seemed like an unattainable goal," Jewel says. "But now I'm living my dream."

Her Best Tip: Jewel varies her workout by taking as many different fitness classes as she can—everything from Tae Bo to core conditioning. She says that mixing up her activities makes it more fun.

Maximum-Results Gym Workout

The truth is out: Real women *do* have muscles, and strength training is an ideal way to blast calories, look more sculpted, and approach life with unparalleled energy. This gym workout by Wayne L. Westcott, Ph.D. CSCS, and Tracy D'Arpino, B.S., LPTA, will give you 16 moves and show you how to employ them in 5 different high-intensity programs. By using a fresh technique every week for 5 weeks, you'll keep strengthening your target muscles in new ways for faster, more effective workouts.

"High-intensity workouts are more time-efficient, typically requiring less than 30 minutes," says Westcott. "They also are more productive, generally resulting in greater strength and muscle gains during a given training period." Fast, effective, and producing unprecedented positive changes in the shape of your body—what could be better than that?

Guidelines: You'll use some or all of the exercises shown in this chapter, changing the order, number of reps, and amount of weight weekly according to the 5 different training techniques that follow. By the end of 5 weeks, you'll have cycled through all 5 high-intensity techniques. Then you'll go back to a traditional strength-training program for 5 weeks, performing 1–2 sets of 8–12 reps of all of the moves shown here (or any total-body strength program of your choice from other chapters). After that period, return to your high-intensity training cycle for another 5 weeks. If you've never worked in this way before, you may want to take 2–3 weeks to master the exercises, performing 1–2 sets of 8–12 reps of each move before starting the amped-up training.

Do each high-intensity program twice a week with at least 2 days of rest between training days (for example, train on Mondays and Fridays).

Warm-up: Begin with 5–10 minutes of low-intensity exercise on any piece of cardio equipment.

Cooldown: End your workout with a static stretch for all of your major muscle groups, holding each stretch for about 30 seconds without bouncing.

Cardio: Get 30–45 minutes of aerobic activity 3–4 times a week on the days that you don't strength train. Make 1 of these days a 30-minute interval workout (for instance, alternate 1–3 minutes of a higher-intensity activity such as running with 1–2 minutes of a lesser-intensity activity such as fast walking or easy jogging).

Ab essentials: Since the moves in this program don't specifically target your abdominal muscles, do 2 sets of 10–20 reps of crunches or any other ab exercise of your choice from Chapter 2: Awesome Abs 3–4 days a week when you do your strength and/or cardio workouts.

Five High-Intensity Training Techniques

You've already learned a couple of these techniques, and now is the time to expand your repertoire. There are 2 basic principles to follow when performing any type of high-intensity training: Rather than adding more exercises or completing more sets, do one of the following:

1. Extend the set with 1 of 3 protocols, which increases volume (called pre-exhaustion, breakdown, and assisted).

2. Extend each rep within a set by slowing the reps down (called negative or positive training).

Any of the following methods will effectively develop muscle tissue. Use each one in the order listed for one week before going on to the next, according to the guidelines above.

Note: For all of these, you'll select a minimum of five moves (one per muscle group) according to the "Selecting Your Moves" instructions (page 285), except when doing the pre-exhaustion technique, for which you'll do all 16 exercises as supersets.

1. Breakdown: As your muscles fatigue, reduce the amount of weight you're using to complete and extend a set.

What to do: Choose a weight amount that allows you to complete 8–10 full repetitions with good form through a full range of motion at a slow speed (2 seconds to lift, 4 seconds to lower) to fatigue. Immediately reduce your weight load by 10–20 percent and complete an additional 2–5 reps. (For example: Do a leg extension using 60 pounds, then reduce to 50 pounds.)

2. Assisted: Train with a partner who can help you complete a few extra repetitions (2–5 reps more) when your muscles become fatigued.

What to do: Perform 8–10 reps with good form through a full range of motion at a slow speed (2 seconds to lift, 4 seconds to lower) to fatigue. Without decreasing weight, continue to perform 2–5 more reps using your own strength, letting your partner assist you through the lifting and lowering phases as needed.

3. Slow-positive emphasis: By slowing down your movement during the lifting phase, you'll place maximum tension on the muscle during its contraction, or shortening, phase.

What to do: Perform 5 reps to fatigue, taking 10 seconds to lift and 4 seconds to lower. Use enough weight to fatigue by the final rep.

4. Slow-negative emphasis: By slowing down your movement during the lowering phase, you're placing maximum tension on the muscle while it is lengthening.

What to do: Perform 5 reps to fatigue, taking 4 seconds for the lifting phase and 10 seconds for the lowering phase. Because it's difficult to control heavy weight as you move slowly through the lengthening (return) segment, you may need to reduce your weight slightly (10–20 percent) for this technique. (Also, since the muscles are lengthening during negative work, you can get much more sore due to more muscle breakdown, which is intended to a reasonable degree. Avoid excessive effort, which can lead to injury.)

5. Pre-exhaustion: To target a specific muscle group, you'll do at least 2 exercises back-to-back without resting in between. You'll start with an isolated move that will "pre-fatigue" the muscle, and finish with a multimuscle exercise that brings in fresh muscles to assist the one you're targeting. (For example: a leg extension to fatigue the quadriceps, followed by a leg press, which still works quadriceps, but also the hamstrings and buttocks.)

What to do: Do exercises 1–14 in the order shown, but in pairs or groups as supersets (Moves 1–3; 4–6; 7–8; 9–10; 11–12; and 13–14).

Note: You may leave out exercises 15 and 16; or alternatively, do Move 15 prior to Move 7, and Move 16 prior to Move 11. For the isolation exercise (first of a pair, or first and second of a group of three), choose a weight allowing you to perform 8–10 reps with good form through a full range of motion at a slow speed (2 seconds to lift, 4 seconds to lower) to full fatigue. Without resting, perform 4–5 good reps of the final exercise, using as much weight as you can (because of muscle fatigue, this will be less weight than if you did the exercises alone).

Selecting Your Moves

The exercises appear in the order necessary to complete the pre-exhaustion program, but for the other 4 regimens, you'll pick at least 1 per category, working larger muscle groups first, such as legs or back (if you choose to do multimuscle). Try to vary between multimuscle and isolation exercises throughout the 5 weeks, using this key. If you choose to focus on isolating body parts, you may need to do more than one exercise.

Legs/Hips/Buttocks:
Isolation: leg extension, seated leg curl, hip abduction, hip adduction
Multimuscle: leg press (or barbell squat), front lunge

Back:
Isolation: pullover, bent-over rear fly
Multimuscle: lat pull-down, seated stack row

Shoulders:
Isolation: lateral raise
Multimuscle: seated shoulder press

Chest:
Isolation: chest cross
Multimuscle: chest press

Arms:
Isolation: biceps curl, triceps cable press-down

The Moves

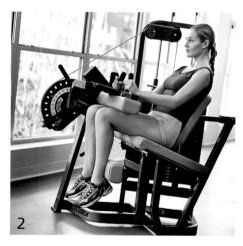

1. Leg extension: Sit with back against pad, knees bent, pad in front of ankles, and feet relaxed; hold handles for support. Straighten legs up in an arc, keeping hips and back against pad (as shown). Return to starting position and repeat.
Weight: 30–60 pounds.
Strengthens quadriceps.

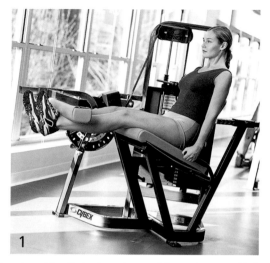

2. Seated leg curl: Sit with legs straight, pad behind ankles, and support pad across thighs; hold handles for support. Keeping back and hips against machine back and seat, bend knees to bring heels down and under seat (as shown). Straighten legs and repeat.
Weight: 40–70 pounds.
Strengthens hamstrings.

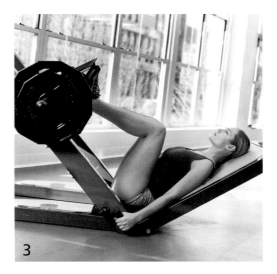

3

3. Leg press: Adjust seat back to a 45-degree angle and sit with feet hip-width apart on center of plate, legs straight but not locked. Keeping back against pad, grasp support handles and unlock plate. Bend knees in toward chest until they're in line with hips (as shown). Straighten legs, pressing through heels, and repeat. (**Note:** You can do a squat with a barbell instead, using 45–90 pounds.)

Weight: Add 25 pounds per side, up to 235 pounds total.

Strengthens quadriceps, hamstrings, and buttocks.

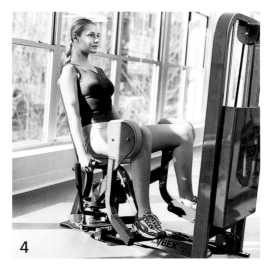

4

4. Hip abduction: Sit with pads close to knees on the outside of thighs; place feet on foot plates with legs slightly apart. Contract abs so that hips are firmly against the back pad and hips are stable. Maintain alignment and press legs out to a comfortable distance (as shown). Return slowly to starting position; repeat.

Weight: 50–70 pounds.

Strengthens upper hips.

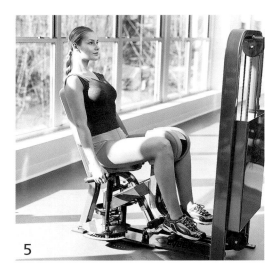

5. Hip adduction: Sit with pads on the inside of thighs at knees; place feet on foot plates with legs slightly more than hip-width apart. Keeping back against pad, contract abs and hold handles for support. Press legs together until they almost touch (as shown). Return to starting position and repeat.

Weight: 60–90 pounds.

Strengthens inner thighs.

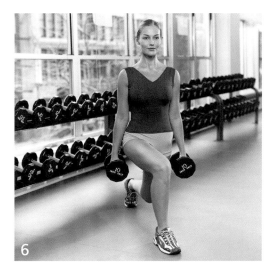

6. Front lunge: Stand with feet hip-width apart, holding a dumbbell in each hand with arms hanging at sides and palms in. Contract abs, bringing spine to a neutral position. Step forward with one foot, keeping torso centered, bending both knees so that front knee aligns with front ankle and back knee approaches the floor, keeping heel lifted (as shown). Push off front foot, stepping back to start. Repeat on one side, then switch legs to complete set.

Weight: 10–20 pounds in each hand.

Strengthens quadriceps, hamstrings, buttocks, and calves.

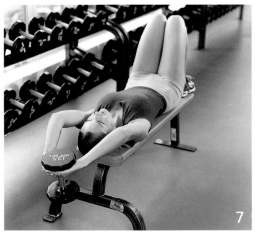

7. Pullover: Lie faceup on a flat bench with knees bent, heels on edge of bench. Hold a single dumbbell vertically with hands clasped, arms extended above midchest, and elbows slightly bent. Draw shoulder blades down and together; maintain elbow position, then bring dumbbell as far behind head as possible without changing torso position, or until upper arms are even with ears (as shown). Return to start by contracting back muscles.

Weight: 12–20 pounds.

Strengthens middle back, upper chest, and shoulders.

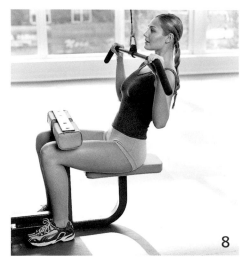

8. Lat pull-down: Grasp a long bar with an overhand grip, arms slightly more than shoulder-width apart, and sit with knees bent, feet flat, and arms extended. Lean back from hips so that bar aligns over chest. Bend elbows in toward waist, keeping wrists in line with elbows (as shown). Straighten arms and repeat.

Weight: 40–90 pounds.

Strengthens middle back, shoulders, and biceps.

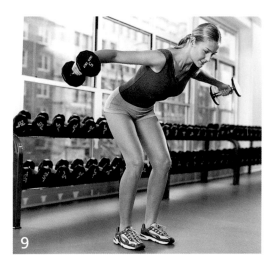

9. Bent-over rear fly: Standing with a dumbbell in each hand, bend knees and flex forward from hips at about a 45-degree angle. Let arms hang in a slight arc in line with shoulders, palms facing in. Using abs to maintain position, lift arms up and out to shoulder height without changing elbow position (as shown). Return to starting position and repeat.

Weight: 5–8 pounds.

Strengthens upper and middle back and rear shoulders.

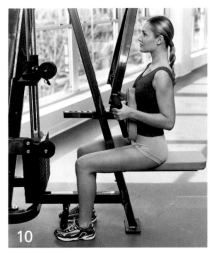

10. Seated stack row: Sit with seat adjusted so that front pad is at upper-rib-cage height; lean lightly on pad and bend knees, keeping feet flat on the floor. Hold vertical handles with arms extended and palms facing in. Squeeze shoulder blades together, then bend elbows back and toward lower rib cage without rocking torso, keeping wrists straight and elbows close to body (as shown). Straighten arms and repeat.

Weight: 40–90 pounds.

Strengthens middle back, rear shoulders, and biceps.

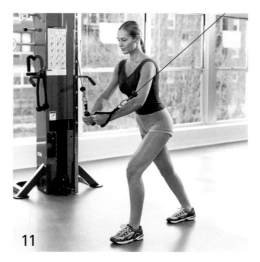

11. Chest cross: Attach handles to upper cables of a high-cable-pulley machine, then stand with one foot in front of the other, holding a handle in each hand, arms open, elbows bent in a slight arc, and palms facing in. Contract abs to maintain neutral spine position; then keeping elbow arc, press arms together until knuckles almost touch (as shown) Release and repeat.

Weight: 20–40 pounds.

Strengthens chest and front shoulders.

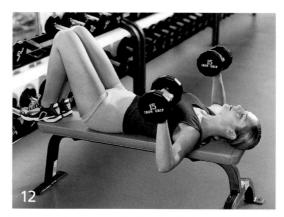

12. Chest press: Lie faceup on a flat bench with knees bent and feet on bench edge. Hold a dumbbell in each hand above midchest with arms straight and palms facing forward (or lie on a bench-press machine, adjusted to 30–60 pounds). Drawing shoulder blades together, bend elbows until even with shoulders, keeping wrists over elbows (as shown). Press up to starting position.

Weight: 15–25 pounds in each hand; 60–90 pounds on bench-press machine.

Strengthens chest, front shoulders, and triceps.

weight-room workouts

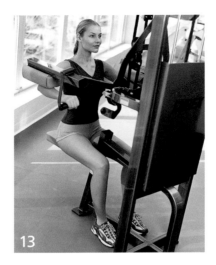

13. Lateral raise: Sit with knees bent and feet flat on the floor. Hold support handles with wrists straight and adjust pads over upper arms and elbows. Lift arms upward to shoulder height using upper arms, not forearms, keeping neck relaxed (as shown). Slowly lower to starting position.

Weight: 20–40 pounds.

Strengthens middle shoulder.

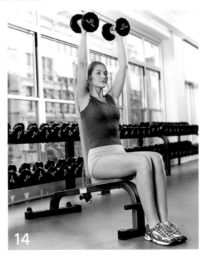

14. Seated shoulder press: Sit on an incline bench adjusted to 90 degrees, holding a dumbbell in each hand at shoulder height with wrists straight, palms in, and elbows bent and close to torso. Contract abs to keep back firmly against back pad. Draw shoulder blades down and together, then press dumbbells up and overhead until arms are straight but not locked (as shown). Slowly lower and repeat.

Weight: 8–15 pounds in each hand.

Strengthens shoulders and upper back.

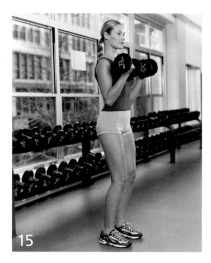

15

15. Biceps curl: Stand with knees slightly bent, holding a dumbbell in each hand with arms hanging by sides and palms facing forward. Contract abs to maintain a neutral spine. Keeping elbows aligned under shoulders, bend elbows to bring dumbbells up and in toward shoulders (as shown). Lower and repeat.

Weight: 5–15 pounds in each hand.
Strengthens biceps.

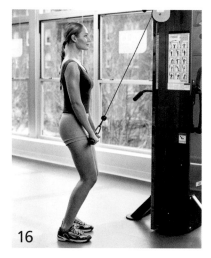

16

16. Triceps cable press-down: Stand facing a high-cable-pulley machine with feet hip-width apart and knees bent; grasp a short bar with an overhand grip. Hold the bar with elbows bent and close to waist, and forearms even with elbows, parallel to each other and the floor. Maintaining shoulder and elbow position, press bar down toward thighs (as shown). Return to starting position and repeat.

Weight: 30–60 pounds.
Strengthens triceps.

weight-room workouts

Weight-Room Etiquette

For newcomers in particular, the atmosphere in many gyms can be intimidating—especially if you forgo the machines for free weights. Here are some rules of the road to make the experience more pleasant:

- Share and share alike. Many people monopolize space, staking their claim with a water bottle while they cross the gym to work on a different body part. Feel free to ask, "Can I work in?" if someone is hogging an area or machine and interfering with your routine.

- Rack your weights. The mantra is, "If you can lift it, you can put it away." Always put bars and dumbbells back in their proper place, and remove weight plates from machines when you've finished your sets.

- Tote a towel. Wipe down equipment after you're through using it, even if you don't see any sweat.

- Don't monopolize the mirror. It's an unspoken rule to not block the view of someone who's scrutinizing the reflection of his or her form. If there's nowhere else to go, ask nicely if that person minds sharing the space.

Ultimate Word

Are you self-conscious because you aren't (yet) as toned and buff as some of the people at your gym? What you wear can help you fit in and give you confidence. "Black or navy are always slimming colors," says Dinah Erasmus, *Shape's* associate fashion editor. She suggests wearing a supportive top with a shelf bra or a sports bra under a fitted T-shirt made of a Lycra blend.

"Baggy or loose clothes don't flatter anyone," says Erasmus. For bottoms, she recommends wearing "a cute, relaxed-fit capri or wide-leg dark pant with side stripes. A vertical stripe is slimming, and wide-leg pants balance out the hips and create a nice, straight line from waist to feet. Again, the key is to use well-constructed fabrics. Nike and Lucy make great bottoms for fuller figures."

The gym might be a fashion show for some people, but once you get into the routine, your gym outfits will be the last thing on your mind. You'll be thinking about how good you feel and how great you're going to look in street clothes.

Now that you have the tools and techniques that allow you to maximize your gym's weight room, we're going to devote the next chapter to workouts that can travel easily from home to the health club, depending on your circumstances and schedule.

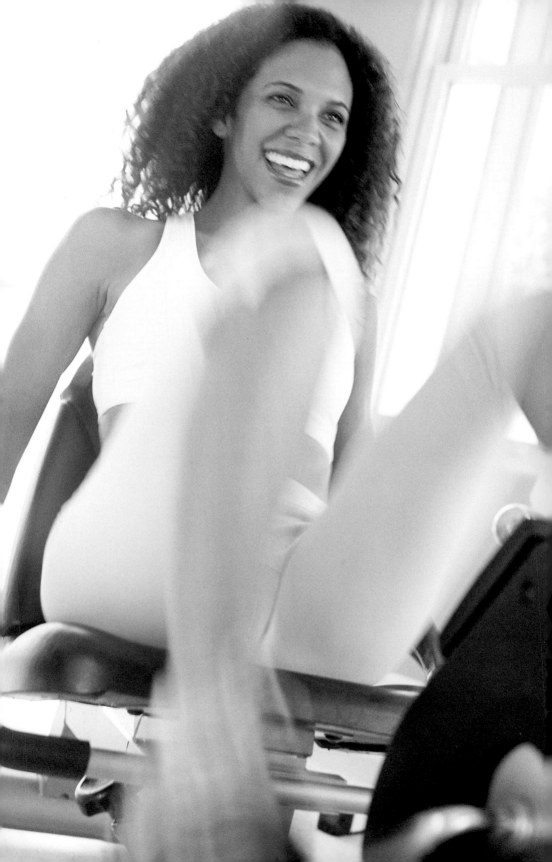

chapter 12

programs for home or gym

When it comes to working on your Ultimate Body, some of you undoubtedly prefer the privacy of your homes—after a hard day's work, the last thing you probably want to do is schlep to the health club and then wait your turn to use the machines. But even if you just can't wait to hit the gym to straighten out your physical and mental kinks, it's nice to have options—and that's what this chapter provides.

This Chapter's To-Do List

In the following pages, you'll learn:

- The pros and cons of home and gym workouts
- A health-club routine with options to do at home— without missing a beat
- A home workout that you can translate to the gym for variation

Are You a Homebody or a Gym Rat?

Answer these questions to learn more about your workout-environment preferences:

1. Are you able to stay motivated exercising by yourself?

2. Are you more likely to work out if you don't have to fight traffic or bad weather?

3. Do you get distracted around other people?

4. Do you feel self-conscious exercising in public?

5. Do you like the flexibility of working out whenever you feel like it?

6. Are you more likely to stick to a schedule if you've paid for a gym membership?

7. Do you like to look around and get inspiration and energy from others?

8. Do you enjoy the social aspect of going to a health club?

9. Do you like using a variety of high-tech machines?

10. Do you appreciate having access to the input of exercise professionals?

If you answered yes to questions 1 through 5, most likely you primarily exercise at home. "Not everyone feels comfortable in the gym environment," confirms Susan Fleck, a certified trainer for Homebodies, an in-home personalized-training company in New York City and Los Angeles. "At home, you can use music and lighting to create an atmosphere that makes you feel good." She also believes that working out at home encourages more creativity. "You have to find ways to make your muscles work hard without the assistance of machines," she explains. "Whether you want to tone your muscles or improve your balance, there's so much you can do just by using your own body weight and dumbbells."

If you answered yes to questions 6 through 10, you'll probably be better served by leaving home most of the time. "The gym has a wide range of equipment options, so you can get more variety in your workouts," says Cheryl Graves, a trainer at Breakthru Fitness in Pasadena, California. "Also, gym machines allow you to add resistance until you reach the point of failure and provide more control than you get with free weights."

Other reasons to hit the road? "The great energy level and potential for social interaction can psych you up and inspire you to train harder," she adds. Plus, you have few distractions at a place dedicated to exercising.

But whether you're a homebody or a gym rat, the goal is usually the same: Get the best possible workout to build strong, beautiful muscles. And even if you really prefer one or the other, you have the option to mix them up—getting your workout in at home if time or bad weather prevents you from going out; or hitting the gym for a change of scenery (and machinery). Our two routines offer the option for going to the gym's weight room and using its equipment, or staying at home with just a pair of dumbbells. Each program consists of moves to strengthen and tone all of your major muscle groups, proving that you can get and stay in great shape, no matter where you choose to train.

Routine One: The Gym Workout with Home Options

This program, created by trainer Cheryl Graves, utilizes machines available in any gym. These exercises challenge your muscles by using more resistance than you can get with dumbbells, while certain machines—like the weight-assisted pull-up/dip apparatus—allow you to do supereffective, muscle-building moves that you might not have the strength to do otherwise.

Guidelines: Do this workout 2–3 times per week, taking a day off in between workouts; review the moves for sets, reps, and weight directions. Rest 30–45 seconds between sets or after each superset. After completing all 6 exercises according to the set guidelines, do 2–3 sets (15 reps per set) of any abdominal exercise (see Chapter 2: Awesome Abs).

To Progress: Once you can do a full set of reps without feeling fatigued, increase the resistance by 10–15 percent, and build up to 25 reps per set of your abdominal exercises.

Warm-up: Begin with 5 minutes on any piece of cardio equipment, programmed at a low intensity; then do one easy set of 10–15 reps on the assisted-pull-up machine adjusted to 70 percent of your body weight.

Cooldown: End your workout with a static stretch for all of your major muscle groups, holding each stretch for about 30 seconds without bouncing.

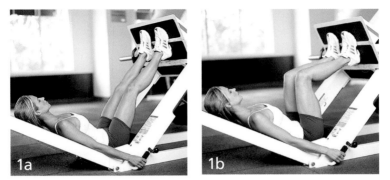

1. Leg press: Adjust the seat of a decline leg-press machine to 45 degrees, then sit with feet hip-width apart and legs straight but not locked. Contract abs, keep back against pad, and grasp handles (a). Release foot locks and bend knees toward chest until they're in line with hips, but no farther (b). Pressing through heels, straighten legs while keeping knees aligned with feet. Slowly return to starting position, then repeat.

Do 3 sets of increasing weight and decreasing reps, as follows:
- Set 1: 25 pounds per side/15 reps.
- Set 2: 30 pounds per side/12 reps.
- Set 3: 45 pounds per side/8–10 reps.

Strengthens quadriceps, hamstrings, and buttocks.

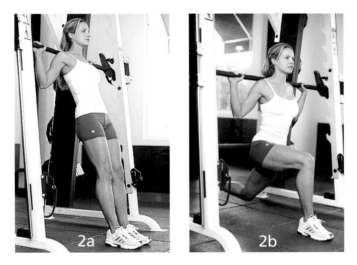

2. Alternating Smith lunges: Standing inside a Smith machine, hold bar across your shoulders with an overhand grip, hands slightly wider than shoulder-width. Position feet slightly in front of bar and contract abs (a). Take a step back with one foot, bending both knees to lower body. Keep front knee in line over front ankle as back knee approaches floor with back heel lifted (b). Push off back foot to return to starting position. Repeat with opposite leg.

Do 3 consecutive sets of 8–12 reps with each leg without resting between sets. Add 1–25 pounds on each side (depending on machine).

Strengthens quadriceps, hamstrings, buttocks, and calves; hip abductors and adductors work as stabilizers.

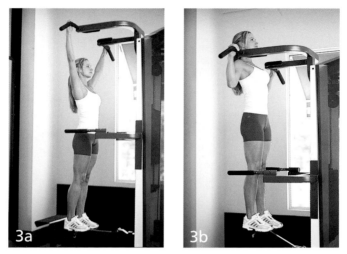

3. Weight-assisted pull-up: Adjust machine to 50–60 percent of your body weight. Stand (or kneel, depending on the machine) on platform with feet (or knees) and hips in line with shoulders. Grasp wide handles with arms extended. Contract abs, lean torso slightly backward, and pull shoulder blades down and back (a). Pull yourself up, driving elbows toward waist while lifting chest up toward handles; finish with elbows pointing down at sides (b). Slowly straighten arms, then repeat.

Do one set (8–12 reps) of this move, followed by one set (8–12 reps) of Move 4. Rest for 30–45 seconds, then repeat for 3 supersets total.

Strengthens upper and middle back, shoulders, and biceps.

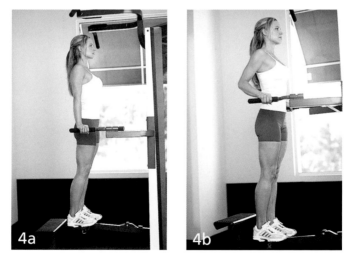

4. Weight-assisted tri-dip: Adjust machine to 50–60 percent of your body weight. Stand or kneel (depending on the machine) on platform and grip lower bars with palms facing in. Allow body weight to move platform down so that arms are straight without being locked (a). Bend elbows to 90 degrees, or as close to parallel to the floor as is comfortable (b), then slowly straighten arms to starting position and repeat.

See Move 3 for set/rep guidelines; go to Move 5 after completing 3 supersets.

Strengthens upper back, shoulders, and triceps.

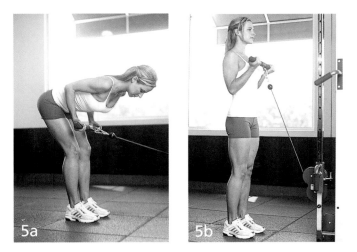

5. Cable combo: Attach a straight bar to low-cable-pulley machine, then stand at arm's length, holding bar with both hands, palms facing up. Separate feet hip-width apart, contract abs, and bend forward from hips until torso is almost parallel to floor. Use back muscles to bend elbows back toward waist (a). Repeat for 8–12 reps.

Do this superset combo a total of 3 times (8–12 reps each time), using 15–40 pounds (adjust weight for each part of exercise).

Strengthens middle back, rear shoulders, and biceps.

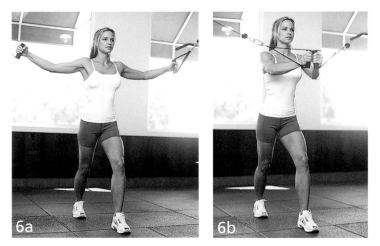

6. Standing cable crossover: Attach a single handle to both high cables inside a cable cage, then stand with a handle in each hand. Stagger feet with one just in front of the other; hip-width apart. Extend arms at shoulder height, palms facing forward, and bend elbows in a slight arc. Lean slightly forward from hips (a). Contract abs and squeeze shoulder blades together, then bring knuckles together in front of chest without changing elbow position (b). Return to starting position, then repeat.

Do 3 sets of increasing weight and decreasing reps, as follows:
- Set 1: 10 pounds/15 reps.
- Set 2: 15 pounds/12 reps.
- Set 3: 15–20 pounds/8–10 reps.

Strengthens front of shoulders, and chest.

The Home Option

This workout variation was developed by certified trainer Susan Fleck of Homebodies. All six moves require concentration and balance, and work multiple muscles at once, just as the gym techniques do. Simple and fun, the exercises train your body in the functional ways that you move in daily life.

Guidelines: Do this workout 2–3 times per week, taking a day off in between workouts; review the moves for set and rep directions. Select a weight based on your strength-training experience: If you've been exercising less than 3 months, use 3- to 5-pound weights; if you've been working at least twice a week for 3–6 months, use 5- to 8-pound weights; if you've been training consistently for 6 months or more, use 8- to 12-pound weights or heavier.

To progress: When you can complete all of the sets and reps, increase weight by 2–3 pounds.

Warm-up: Begin your workout with 5–10 minutes of low- to moderate-intensity cardio activity, such as jumping rope, walking briskly, or climbing stairs.

Cooldown: End with 5–10 minutes more of cardio activity, then stretch all of your major muscle groups, holding each stretch for about 30 seconds without bouncing.

Misstep:

Trying to go it entirely alone. Regardless of whether you opt to work out at home or at the gym, consider having a few sessions with a personal trainer to get you on the right track. A fitness professional can help you learn effective, safe form whether you're working with free weights or on machines. If you belong to a gym, you'll probably be able to find someone there. You should ask friends for a referral, but if you draw a blank, you can go to the Website of the American Council on Exercise **(http://acefitness.org)** and find someone in your area who's been certified by that organization.

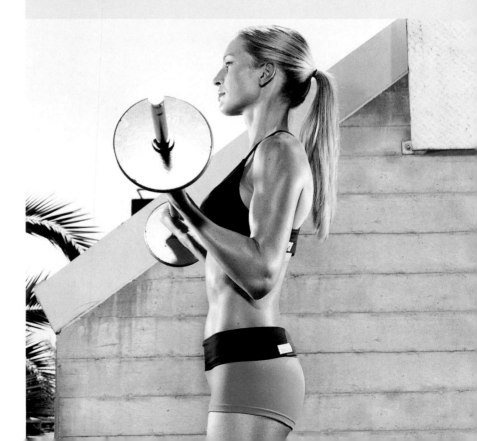

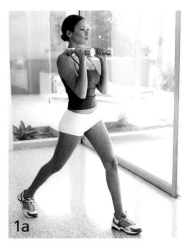

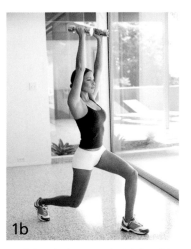

1. Lunge and press: Grasp a dumbbell in each hand, then stand with feet hip-width apart, one foot a full stride in front of the other, and back heel lifted. Hold weights in front of shoulders with elbows bent and close to torso, palms facing in, and abs contracted (a). Bend knees, lowering hips toward floor and keeping front knee in line with ankle, back knee pointing downward. At the same time, straighten arms and press dumbbells overhead (b). Straighten legs as you lower dumbbells to starting position.

Do 12–15 reps, then switch legs and repeat.

Strengthens quadriceps, hamstrings, buttocks, calves, upper back, and shoulders.

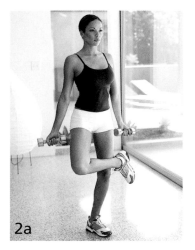

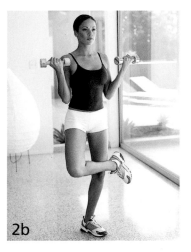

2. Biceps balance: Grasp a dumbbell in each hand with arms hanging by your sides, elbows aligned under shoulders, and palms facing forward. Keeping left knee straight, place right ankle across left thigh so that right knee turns outward with tailbone pointed down and abs contracted (if you're a beginner, lean back against a wall for balance) (a). Maintain this position as you bend both elbows to curl dumbbells toward shoulders (b). Slowly lower dumbbells and repeat for 12–15 reps, then switch sides and repeat.

Strengthens biceps; all leg muscles act as stabilizers.

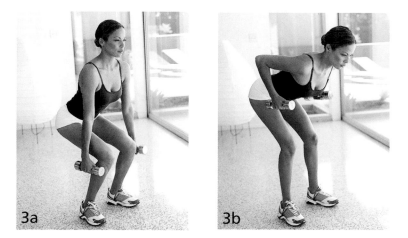

3. Squat combo: Grasp a dumbbell in each hand, and stand with feet hip-width apart, legs straight but not locked, arms handing by sides, and palms facing in. Contract abs and maintain a natural curve in back. Bend both knees, lowering hips until thighs are just about parallel to floor (a). Straighten legs and repeat for 12–15 reps. On the final rep, hold the squat position, bend forward from hips while keeping back flat, and bend both elbows back and up toward your waist; do a "row" for 12–15 reps (b).

Do this superset a total of 2–3 times, resting 30 seconds between supersets.

Strengthens quadriceps, hamstrings, buttocks, middle back, rear shoulders, and biceps.

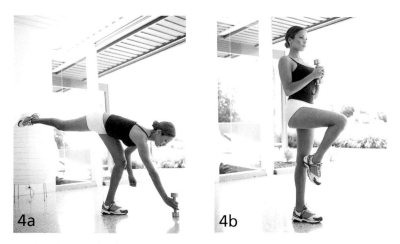

4. One-leg reach: Place a dumbbell upright on the floor, then stand about arm's distance away with feet hip-width apart. Bend forward at hips and balance on left leg while extending right leg behind you, in line with torso. Continue to bend until back is parallel to the floor and reach for the weight with one or both hands (a). Pick up weight and bend elbows to lift it toward chest. Return to upright position, contracting abs while bringing right knee up in front of body to hip height (b). Lower leg to floor and repeat from the beginning, this time placing weight back on the floor (alternately pick up and set down weight with each rep).

Do 12–15 reps, then repeat with opposite leg.

Strengthens quadriceps, hamstrings, buttocks, abdominals, back extensors, middle back, and shoulders.

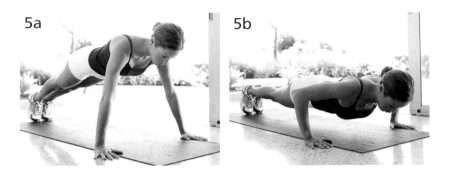

5. Push-up: Kneel on the floor and place hands underneath shoulders, arms straight. Either extend legs so that you're supported on hands and balls of feet, or place knees on the floor behind hips. Contract abs so that your body forms a straight line from head to heels (or knees) (a). Maintain this position while bending elbows to lower chest toward floor until elbows are even with shoulders (b). Push back up to starting position and repeat.

Do a total of 2–3 sets (12–15 reps each), resting 30 seconds between sets. Strengthens chest, front of shoulders, and triceps.

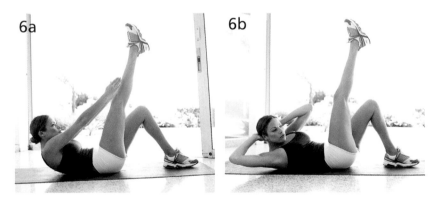

6. Ab challenge: Lie faceup with left knee bent, left foot flat on the floor, right leg extended straight up (in line with hip), and arms by sides. Contract abs to bring spine in contact with the floor. Use abs to lift head, neck, and shoulder blades up, extending arms toward right toes (a). Lower head and arms (arms return to sides) while keeping leg up, and repeat for 15 reps. Rest for 30 seconds, then do another 15 reps with hands behind head, rotating left shoulder toward right knee (b). Switch legs and arms, lifting arms to left toes for 15 reps, then rotating right shoulder to left knee for 15 reps.

Do one set (15 reps) of each portion of the exercise on each side. Strengthens abdominals.

Her Ultimate Turning Point

When Randi Chapin of Pennsylvania tried on her husband's extra-large T-shirt and found it snug, she decided that it was time to lose weight. She started the process by eating better and installing a stair-climber in her bedroom, which she worked out on 3 days a week before work. "I knew if I put it off until later in the day, I'd find an excuse to skip it," she explains.

After losing 20 pounds in 4 months, Randi got bored with the stair-climber and joined the YMCA, where she started weight training and took cardio classes, such as step aerobics and cycling. She soon realized that her new program had another benefit: more energy.

"Instead of coming home and taking a nap, I couldn't wait to get to the gym," she says. Two years later Randi was 80 pounds lighter and loving her 120-pound body.

Her Best Tip: Don't get stuck doing the same workout day in and day out. Switch your workouts every 4–6 weeks for the best results.

Routine Two: The Home Workout with Gym Option

Jennifer Spencer of Canyon Ranch Health Resort & Spa in Tucson, Arizona, devised these 6 supereffective body-sculpting moves to do with very little equipment.

Guidelines: Do this workout 2–3 times per week. Unless otherwise noted, perform 1–3 sets of 8–12 reps if you're using heavier weights to develop strength, and 12–15 reps with lighter weights to build endurance. (Your muscles should always feel challenged by the last 2 reps of each set; as you progress, switch to heavier weights or add more reps.) Rest 1 minute between sets. After completing all 6 exercises, do 2 sets (20–25 reps per set) of any 2 abdominal exercises (see Chapter 2: Awesome Abs).

To Progress: Once you can do a full set of reps without feeling fatigued, increase the resistance by 10–15 percent, and build up to 25 reps per set of your abdominal exercises.

Warm-up: Begin with 5 minutes of light cardio such as marching in place, alternating lunges, or climbing stairs; followed by leg swings (front and back and side-to-side across your body), torso twists, arm swings (front and back), and arm reaches (side-to-side across your body while squatting).

Cooldown: End your workout with 12–16 torso twists, then stretch all of your major muscle groups, holding each stretch for about 30 seconds without bouncing.

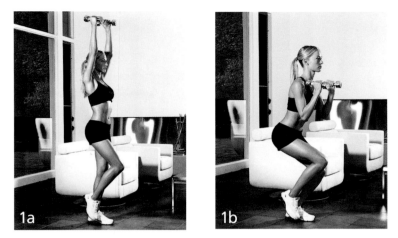

1. One-legged overhead press with mini-squats: Stand with legs straight and feet hip-width apart, holding a dumbbell in each hand in front of shoulders with elbows close to sides and palms in. Lift right foot a few inches off the floor, left knee slightly bent; contract abs and press arms overhead (a). Lower arms to shoulders, then bend left knee, lowering hips to a quarter-squat (b). Straighten left leg with right foot still lifted and repeat combo to complete reps. Switch legs and repeat on opposite side for one set.

Weight: 5- to 8-pound dumbbells.

Strengthens quadriceps, hamstrings, buttocks, shoulders, and upper back; abdominals and spine extensors act as stabilizers.

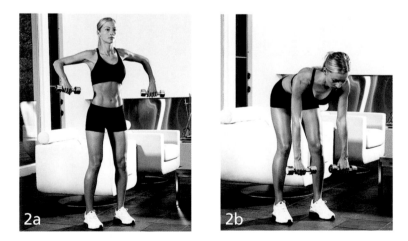

2. Wide-row/dead-lift combo: Stand with feet hip-width apart, holding a dumbbell in each hand, arms hanging at sides, palms facing in, and legs straight but not locked. Squeeze shoulder blades down and together and contract abs while bending and lifting elbows up and out to shoulder height (a). Straighten arms; then, keeping legs straight and lower back naturally curved, bend forward at hips, letting arms hang in front of legs and lowering torso until you feel a stretch in hamstrings (b). Contract buttocks and hamstrings while lifting torso to an upright position and repeat combo.

Weight: 8- to 10-pound dumbbells.

Strengthens shoulders, upper back, buttocks, and hamstrings; abdominals and spine extensors act as stabilizers.

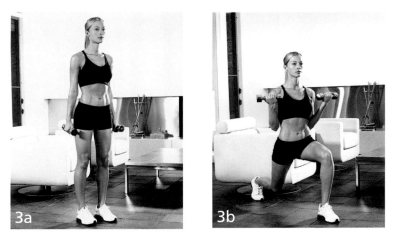

3. Rear-lunge/biceps-arm combo: Stand with feet hip-width apart, holding a dumbbell in each hand, arms at sides, palms in, chest lifted, and abs tight (a). Step back with right foot, bending both knees so that left knee aligns with ankle, right knee approaches the floor with right heel lifted; simultaneously bend elbows, rotating palms up while curling dumbbells toward shoulders (b). Lower arms to your sides and step forward to starting position. Repeat on left side to complete one rep.

Weight: 5- to 8-pound dumbbells.

Strengthens quadriceps, hamstrings, buttocks, calves, biceps, and middle shoulders.

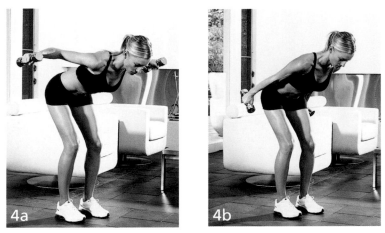

4. Bent-over kickback/rear-fly combo: Stand with feet hip-width apart, holding a dumbbell in each hand, arms bent with elbows at sides, palms in, and forearms parallel to floor. Keeping abs tight, bend knees and bend forward at the hips until torso is almost parallel to the floor, allowing elbows to move forward until pointing at the floor. Maintain position and lift arms up and out to shoulder height, keeping elbows bent (a). Bring elbows back in, aligning upper arms against sides of torso, and immediately straighten both arms behind you without locking elbows (b). Bend elbows back to 90 degrees and, still bent forward, repeat combo.

Weight: 3- to 5-pound dumbbells.

Strengthens rear shoulders, middle back, and triceps.

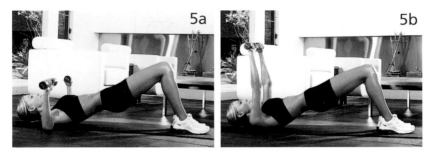

5. Bridge/chest-press combo: Lie faceup on floor with knees bent and feet flat. Hold a dumbbell in each hand with arms bent at 90 degrees, elbows aligned with shoulders, forearms parallel, and palms facing forward. Contract abs, then lift hips until your body forms a line from shoulders to knees (a). Maintain lifted position and straighten arms above midchest without locking elbows (b). Bend elbows and repeat press 4–6 times before lowering hips. Immediately repeat combo to complete 1 set.

Weight: 5- to 10-pound dumbbells.

Strengthens chest, front shoulders, triceps, buttocks, and hamstrings; abdominals, spine extensors, upper hips, and inner thighs act as stabilizers.

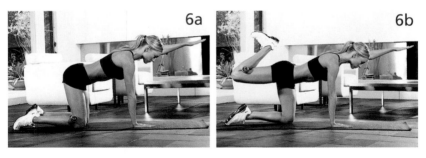

6. Kneeling leg-lift balance: Kneel on all fours with wrists under shoulders and knees under hips. Place a dumbbell behind right knee and squeeze calf against it to hold it in place. Contract abs, extend left arm forward in line with shoulder (a), and then lift right knee up to hip height, foot pressing toward the ceiling, without arching back (b). Lower knee, keeping it slightly off the floor, and repeat leg lifts for all reps with left arm still raised. Repeat with right arm raised and left leg lifting to complete one set.

Weight: 5- to 8-pound dumbbells.

Strengthens hamstrings and buttocks; abdominals and spine extensors act as stabilizers.

The Gym Option

If you have the time and inclination to go to the weight room, these 5 moves will keep you toned and trim. Simply follow the guidelines, warm-up, and cooldown in the home version; and you'll be good to go.

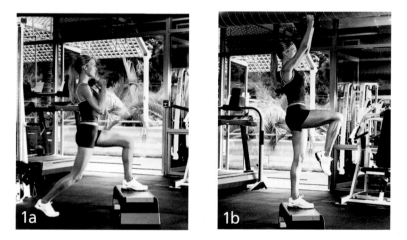

1. Step-up balance/overhead press: Holding a dumbbell in each hand, stand facing an 8- to 10-inch bench or step with weights in front of shoulders and elbows close to sides. Placing left foot on bench, bend both knees, keeping left knee aligned with ankle and right heel lifted (a). Push off right foot to lift yourself up onto the bench, straightening left leg while bending right knee to hip height in front of you; simultaneously straighten arms overhead (b). Lower dumbbells to shoulder height and step down with right foot, then left. Repeat combo on opposite side, placing right foot on bench to complete one rep.

Weight: 5- to 8-pound dumbbells.

Strengthens quadriceps, hamstrings, buttocks, calves, shoulders, and upper back; abdominals and spine extensors act as stabilizers.

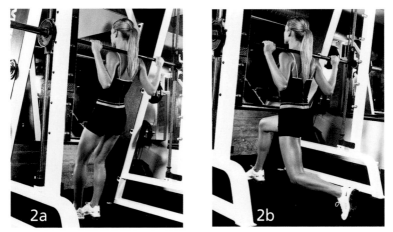

2. Smith lunge: Adjust the bar of a Smith machine to shoulder height, then stand in the center with upper shoulders against the bar. Hold bar with an overhand grip slightly wider than shoulder-width apart and unlock the bar. Then walk both feet about one foot ahead of the bar, hip-width apart, with legs straight but not locked and abs drawn in (a). Keeping chest lifted, step backward with left foot into a lunge, bending both knees so that right knee aligns with ankle and left knee approaches the floor with left heel lifted (b). Push back to starting position and repeat with right leg back to complete one rep. Complete all reps.

Weight: 0–20 pounds on each side, depending on machine.
Strengthens quadriceps, hamstrings, buttocks, and calves.

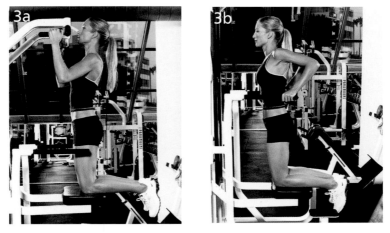

3. Pull-up and dip: Adjust a pull-up machine to 40–60 percent of your body weight, then stand or kneel on the movement pad (depending on machine) as you grasp the handles with palms in. Allow your weight to move pad downward so that arms are straight but not locked. Bend elbows to pull yourself up so that chin is above bar (a). Lower and repeat for 8–12 reps. Next, place hands on the dip bars, palms in and slightly behind shoulders, lowering yourself so that upper arms are close to parallel to the floor (b). Press downward on the dip bars while straightening arms and repeat for 8–12 reps. (Completing both exercises equals one set.)
Strengthens middle back, rear shoulders, biceps, and triceps.

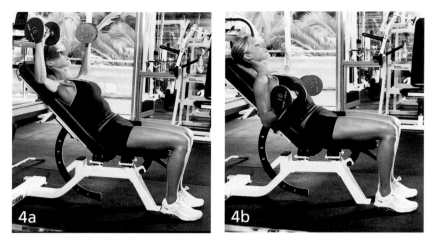

4. Incline press and curl: Adjust an incline bench to 45 degrees and sit back on bench, holding a dumbbell in each hand close to chest with knees bent and feet flat. Contract abs, bringing back in contact with bench, and extend arms above midchest, hands up and palms facing forward. Bend elbows until aligned with shoulders (a). Straighten arms over chest and repeat for 8–12 reps. Next, lower arms to hang by sides in line with shoulders, hands down, and palms forward. Maintaining arm position, bend elbows, curling dumbbells up toward shoulders (b). Lower and repeat for 8–12 reps. (Completing both exercises equals one set.)

Weight: 8- to 10-pound dumbbells.

Strengthens chest, front shoulders, triceps, and biceps.

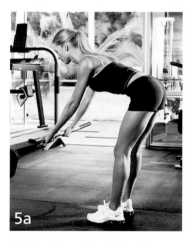
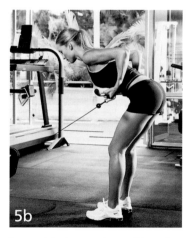

5. Bent-knee dead-lift cable row: Attach a straight bar to a low-cable pulley, then grasp bar with an underhand grip, hands slightly more than shoulder-width apart. Stand farther than an arm's length from the machine, feet hip-width apart and knees slightly bent. Extend arms down toward thighs. Keeping back straight and abs contracted, bend forward from hips until you feel hamstrings stretch (a). Contract back muscles and bend elbows back and up, bringing bar toward lower rib cage (b). Straighten arms, then contract buttocks and hamstrings to stand upright; repeat combo.

Weight: 25–40 pounds.

Strengthens middle back, rear shoulders, buttocks, and hamstrings; abdominals and spine extensors act as stabilizers.

Q. I exercise 12 hours a week, including swimming, trail running, and yoga. Do I really need to strength train, too? If so, what's the minimum amount that I can get away with?

A. "Even though you're already really active, you're leaving out a crucial component of exercise that has far-reaching ramifications as you age," warns Kent Adams, Ph.D., CSCS, an associate professor at the University of Louisville in Kentucky. Research suggests that endurance exercises such as jogging or swimming aren't sufficient for maintaining muscle mass—only strength training can do the job. And while a weight-bearing exercise such as trail running can help maintain bone density in the spine and hips, combining this type of exercise with strength work can help even more.

You can reap the benefits of weight training in just 15–20 minutes of doing a total-body regimen twice a week, using dumbbells at home. "The key is lifting heavy enough weights that you come close to failure on your last repetition," Adams explains. "If you're doing 8 reps, it needs to be a true 8." This is especially important if you're performing just 1 set of each exercise.

Not only will strength training benefit you later in life, but "it will have tremendous benefits for the other activities you love to do right now," says Adams.

Ultimate Word

Just because you're heading out of town doesn't mean that your healthy habits have to fall by the wayside. Those of you who mostly work out at home have no excuse: You can probably continue your usual routine by toting your paraphernalia with you and continuing to exercise at your destination. If you prefer a gym routine, check these directory-based Websites to help you stay on track—no matter where you trek or what you like to do.

- **healthclubs.com** for gyms galore. Many belong to the International Health, Racquet, and Sportsclub Association (IHRSA) Passport Program, which gives members of participating clubs guest privileges in over 3,000 clubs worldwide when traveling.

- **active.com** to find year-round runs, walks, and events, including classes in parks and community centers at your destination.

- **yogafinder.com** to find a yoga class or teacher almost anywhere in the world.

There's only one factor left that might be keeping you from achieving your Ultimate Body: what you're eating. In the next chapter, we'll give you the most important information on eating healthfully in order to stay fit and look great.

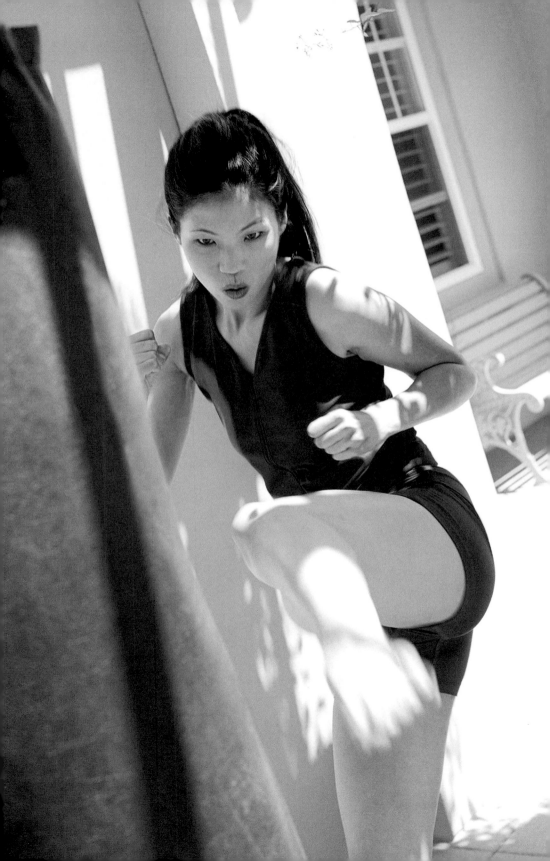

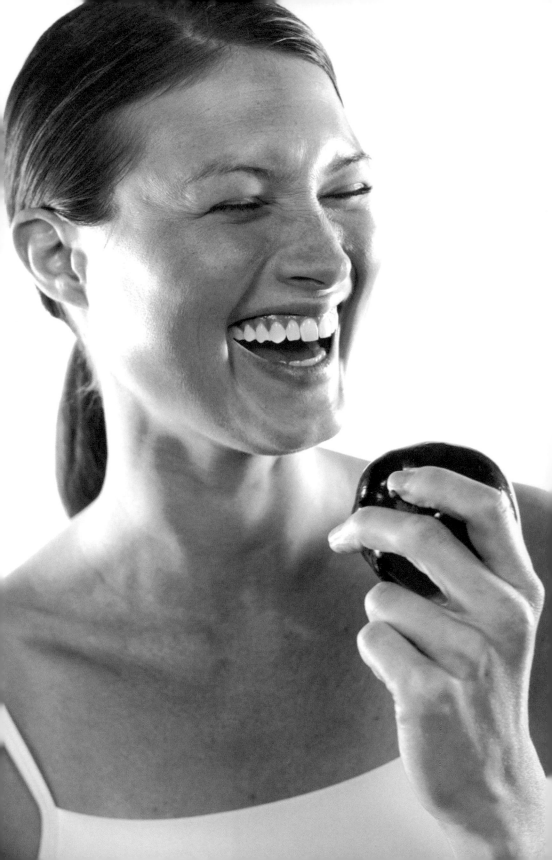

chapter 13

eat smart, eat lean

One of the crucial elements in achieving your Ultimate Body is good nutrition. Eating right will help you lose weight and gain the energy that you need to fuel your workouts. Following our guidelines will not only help you drop pounds and feel great, but can also cut your risk for heart disease, some types of cancer, osteoporosis, diabetes, and arthritis.

This Chapter's To-Do List

In the following pages, you'll learn:

- Kitchen makeovers that will support your efforts to eat healthfully

- Shopping strategies for healthful, low-fat, high-fiber foods that are also appetizing

- Fabulous low-fat cooking techniques

- The way to eat for maximum energy

- How to calculate your calorie needs

- Ways to put it all together with great-tasting recipes

Make Over Your Kitchen

Answer yes or no to the following questions:

1. Is your kitchen "white" (stocked with white flour, white rice, white sugar)?

2. Do you know the best picks in the dairy case at the grocery store?

3. When it comes to nutrition, which veggies offer the biggest bang for the buck?

4. Have you banished all fats from your kitchen?

5. Do you have the tools and gadgets you need to cook healthfully?

You should have answered no to questions 1 and 4; and yes to the rest. If you didn't (and even if you did), get ready to give your kitchen an extreme makeover. Now we don't mean the kind that involves sprucing up cabinets, getting a new refrigerator, and replacing drawer handles—it's what's behind the cabinet doors and inside the fridge that really counts. After all, when healthful foods are easily accessible, you'll be more likely to grab them. Owning the tools and appliances that make your life easier and your eating more nutritious leads to better fuel for your Ultimate Body—and possessing the know-how to put it all to good use means that not only will you lose weight, but you'll feel in control of your eating as well.

If your quest for the Ultimate Body includes losing weight and eating healthfully, your kitchen is the true starting point for all of your efforts, and unless you've stocked the right amounts and types of foods, utensils, and gadgets, you're unwittingly undermining yourself. Some of the worst diet saboteurs are lurking right in your own pantry and fridge. Replace these foods with their healthier, lower-fat, and higher-fiber counterparts, and you'll find that weight-loss success will come much more easily.

Remember, if you don't have poor food choices available, you won't be tempted to eat them. Here are the most important things to toss and replace with healthier alternatives.

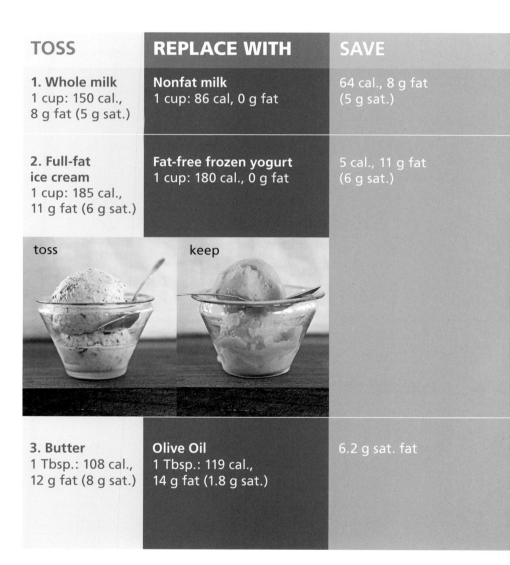

TOSS	REPLACE WITH	SAVE
1. Whole milk 1 cup: 150 cal., 8 g fat (5 g sat.)	**Nonfat milk** 1 cup: 86 cal, 0 g fat	64 cal., 8 g fat (5 g sat.)
2. Full-fat ice cream 1 cup: 185 cal., 11 g fat (6 g sat.)	**Fat-free frozen yogurt** 1 cup: 180 cal., 0 g fat	5 cal., 11 g fat (6 g sat.)
toss keep		
3. Butter 1 Tbsp.: 108 cal., 12 g fat (8 g sat.)	**Olive Oil** 1 Tbsp.: 119 cal., 14 g fat (1.8 g sat.)	6.2 g sat. fat

TOSS	REPLACE WITH	SAVE
4. Full-fat cheese 1 oz.: 93 cal., 7 g fat (4 g sat.)	**Reduced-fat cheese** 1 oz.: 80 cal., 3–5 g fat (2–3 g sat.)	13 cal., 2–4 g fat (1–2 g sat.)
5. Mayonnaise 1 Tbsp.: 100 cal., 11 g fat (2 g sat.)	**Light mayonnaise** 1 Tbsp.: 50 cal., 5 g fat (1 g sat.)	50 cal., 6 g fat (1 g sat.)
6. Potato chips 1 oz.: 152 cal., 10 g fat (3 g sat), 1 g fiber	**Light microwave popcorn** 3-1/2 cups: 70 cal., 1 g fat (0 g sat), 3 g fiber	82 cal., 9 g fat (3 g sat.) *gain* 2 g fiber

toss — keep

TOSS	REPLACE WITH	SAVE
7. White bread 1 slice: 65 cal., 1 g fat, <1 g fiber	**Whole-grain bread** 1 slice: 70 cal., <1 g fat, 3 g fiber	<1 g fat, *gain* 3 g fiber
8. Salad dressing 1 Tbsp.: 69–100 cal.,7–14 g fat (1 g sat.)	**Light or fat-free salad dressing** 1 Tbsp.: 25–35 cal.,0–3 g fat (0 g sat.)	44–65 cal., 7–11 fat (1 g sat.)

TOSS	REPLACE WITH	SAVE
9. White-flour (semolina) pasta 1 cup: 197 cal., 1 g fat; 2 g fiber	**Whole-wheat pasta** 1 cup: 174 cal., 1 g fat; 6 g fiber 20 cal.,	*gain* 4 g fiber
10. White rice ½ cup: 103 cal., 0 g fat, 0 g fiber	**Brown rice** ½ cup: 108 cal., 1 g fat (0 g sat.), 2 g fiber	*gain* 1 g fat, 2 g fiber
11. Soda 1 cup: 101 cal., 0 g fat	**Half orange juice/half seltzer water** 1 cup: 11 cal., 0 g fat	90 cal.
12. Bologna 1 oz.: 89 cal., 8 g fat (3 g sat.)	**Oven-roasted turkey breast** 1 oz.: 38 cal., <1 g fat (<1 g sat.)	51 cal., 7 g fat (>2 g sat.)

toss

keep

| **13. Sugary cereal** 1 cup: 160 cal., 0 g fat, 0 g fiber | **Whole-grain cereal** 1 cup: 147 cal., 1 g fat (0 g sat.), 13 cal., 4 g fiber | *gain* 1 g fat, 4 g fiber |

eat smart, eat lean

TOSS	REPLACE WITH	SAVE
14. Ground beef (70–85% lean) 3 oz.: 231 cal., 21 g protein, 16 g fat (6 g sat.)	**Chicken or turkey breast** 3 oz.: 140 cal., 26 g protein, 3 g fat (<1 g sat.)	91 cal., 13 g fat (> 5 g sat.) *gain* 5 g protein
15. Packaged pastries (e.g., Twinkies) 1: 160 cal., 5 g fat (2 g sat.), 0 g fiber	**Fat-free cookies (e.g., Fig Newtons)** 1: 50 cal., 0 g fat, 1 g fiber	110 cal., 5 g fat (2 sat.) *gain* 1 g fiber

Having a supply of healthy foods on hand is essential to any weight-loss plan, so we're providing you with a low-fat, high-nutrient shopping list that will make it easier to stick to low-calorie meals and snacks and get the daily nutrients you need. When you have nutritious food in your home, you're likely to use it for cooking meals and for snacks. After all, if you don't keep greasy chips and cookies in your cupboard, then you'll probably reach for the whole-grain crackers and reduced-fat peanut butter or a piece of fruit instead.

You'll also be happy to discover that shopping for a healthful, more plant-based diet is often less expensive than loading up on traditional staples like red meat, butter, cheese, sugary cereals, and processed snacks—so grab a cart!

Here's how to stock your kitchen with the best choices that the grocery store has to offer. Listed under each food group, you'll find the reasons why you need to eat these foods, the number of daily servings you should have, and the best picks (including some brand names to look for).

The Produce Section

Research has shown that a diet rich in fruit and vegetables can help manage your weight. Plus, there are hundreds of phytochemicals (natural, protective chemicals found in plant food) in produce, which helps prevent cancer, heart disease, age-related blindness, birth defects, and diabetes. Eat as wide a variety as possible, but especially concentrate on the darker colors, since they tend to contain the most phytochemicals. Servings can be fresh, frozen, dried, and (in some cases) juiced. Canned goods are fine, too, as long as you read the labels to ensure there isn't too much added salt and sugar.

Best Picks:

Fruit:

kiwi

apples

apricots

cantaloupe and honeydew melons

oranges and calcium-fortified orange juice, pink grapefruit, lemons, and limes

berries (such as strawberries, blueberries, and raspberries)

papaya

bananas

red grapes

tomatoes and tomato juice

avocados

Vegetables:

summer and winter squash

greens (such as collard, Swiss chard, spinach, and kale)

broccoli or broccoli rabe

red lettuce

cucumber

bell peppers

roasted red peppers (available in jars)

garlic (fresh)

onions

baby carrots

potatoes

yams

fresh herbs (such as cilantro, basil, and parsley)

pesto (containers of fresh sauce, such as Buitoni)

The Whole-Grain Aisles: Bread, Cereal, and Grains

Choose whole grains over refined products such as white rice and flour, and you'll get more fiber, vitamins, minerals, and phytochemicals. All of these help with weight management and reduce the risk of heart disease, cancer, and diabetes. Read the labels carefully: The first ingredient should be whole grain, whole wheat, or rye (plain or fortified-wheat flour is not whole grain).

Best Picks:

Breakfast Cereals:
Kellogg's All-Bran

General Mills Total

Quaker Oats
(old-fashioned or quick-cooking)

Eggo whole-grain frozen waffles

Grains:
quick-cooking brown rice

buckwheat groats (kasha)

quinoa

whole-wheat and corn tortillas

reduced-fat Triscuits

whole-wheat pasta

whole-wheat flour

Bread:
Pepperidge Farm

Natural Whole Grain

Sara Lee whole wheat

any brand with no more than 90 calories
    and at least 2 grams of fiber per slice

The Fish Counter

Fish is an excellent source of protein: It has all the nutrients of meat, but without the saturated fat. Plus, many varieties of fish are loaded with omega-3 fatty acids, which helps fend off heart disease.

Best Picks:
fresh salmon fillets
water-packed, canned salmon
fresh bluefin or yellowfin tuna
water-packed, canned tuna
fresh king-mackerel fillet
fresh trout

The Bean (Legume) Bins

Beans provide a bounty of dietary fiber, which makes you feel full faster and keeps you from getting hungry again too soon, because it digests slowly. These powerhouses also provide lots of folic acid, a nutrient essential to women of child-bearing age for the development of a healthy baby. Peanuts are from the same family as beans—that is, legumes, which are the edible seeds of plants.

Best Picks:
black beans
kidney beans
pinto beans
garbanzo beans (chickpeas)
white beans
green beans (canned)
reduced-fat peanut butter

The Meat and Poultry Counter

Meat is a good source of protein, iron, and zinc. Cuts with "loin" in the name are often the leanest; but even with these, still trim any visible fat before cooking. Don't be fooled by packaged ground turkey—it often contains more fat than lean ground beef, so check the labels carefully.

Best Picks:
skinless chicken breast
skinless turkey breast
pork tenderloin
lean cuts of beef (such as round steak or sirloin)

The Dairy (and Soy) Case

Milk, yogurt, and cheese offer bone-strengthening calcium and vitamin D, but dairy products also have a lot of saturated fat—even reduced-fat (2 percent) milk. Stick to nonfat or low-fat (1 percent) products, or replace dairy with calcium- and vitamin D-enriched soy products. Soy has plant estrogens that may reduce the risk of some kinds of breast and ovarian cancer.

Best Picks:
skim milk
low-fat yogurt
reduced-fat cheddar cheese
Parmesan cheese
low-fat ice cream or frozen yogurt
enriched soy milk
soy yogurt
soy cheese
soy turkey
fresh or frozen soybeans (edamame)
tofu
eggs
egg whites (packaged and refrigerated)

Nuts, Seeds, and Oils

These products are high in fat, but it's the beneficial kind: monounsaturated fat that helps raise our good cholesterol (HDL) without increasing the bad (LDL). Buy raw, unsalted nuts and keep them in the refrigerator; and get 8-ounce bottles of oil so that you can finish them before they go rancid.

Fat should make up less than 30 percent of your total calories, and less than 10 percent of that should come from saturated fat. Trans fats, found in fast foods and prepared baked goods, should be kept to a minimum—or better yet, eliminated altogether. Starting in 2006, manufacturers will be obligated to list trans fats on food labels. In the meantime, the words *hydrogenated* or *partially hydrogenated fat* will clue you in to their presence.

Best Picks:
almonds, blanched
walnuts, shelled
tahini (sesame-seed paste)
flaxseed
nut butters
olive oil
canola oil
olives
avocados

The Condiment Shelves

Your low-fat cooking will be enhanced by these flavor boosters.

Best Picks:
salt
pepper
fat-free salad dressings
fat-free mayonnaise
ground spices
fresh herbs
flavored vinegars
mustards
low-fat chicken or vegetable broth
salsa
fresh gingerroot
unsweetened-cocoa powder
brown sugar
maple syrup

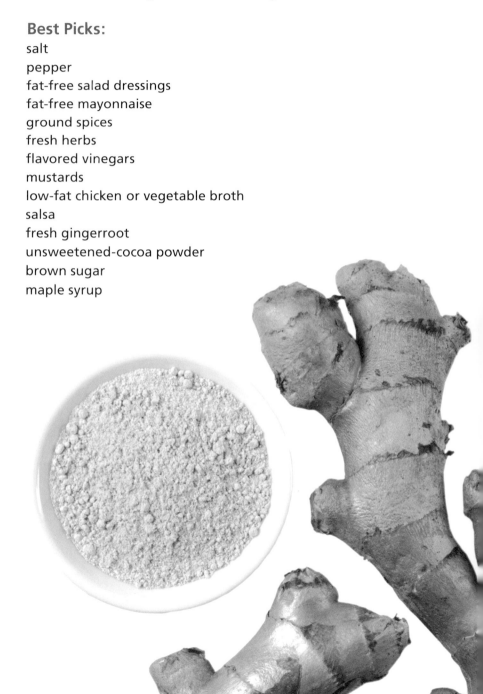

Her Ultimate Turning Point

When Bonnie Camm delivered twin boys prematurely (she already had a 2-year-old at home), good eating went by the wayside. By the time the twins were 4, Bonnie's convenience diet of burgers and fries had caused her weight to soar to 160 pounds—and that's when she realized that she had to make some changes.

She recruited her husband, and they began keeping an eating record. "I was surprised to see how much junk food, mostly cookies and soda, I nibbled on without even realizing it," she says. She made fruits, vegetables, whole grains, and lean meats the centerpiece of her new eating plan and added cardio. Within a year, she'd dropped 45 pounds—and her husband lost 80!

Her Best Tip: Stock up on vegetables and lean cuts of meat when they're on sale and freeze them so that you'll always have the makings of healthy meals on hand.

Make Over Your Menu

So now that your pantry and refrigerator are fully stocked with low-fat, nutritious food, you'll want to make sure that you're putting all those goodies to their ultimate good use.

Here's how to get your daily (or weekly) quota of healthful foods:

- **Produce:** You need 10 servings of fruits and vegetables a day. Does that sound like a lot? It really isn't, when you consider that a serving is one piece of fruit, 1 cup of raw vegetables, ½ cup canned or cooked fruits and vegetables, 1 ounce of dried fruit, or 6 ounces of juice. If you have 2 servings at breakfast, you've already made a good start on the day.

- **Whole grains:** It's easier than you think to get your daily ration of 8 to 10 servings, since a serving is 1 slice of bread; ½ an English muffin, hamburger bun, or bagel; 1 tortilla; ½ cup cooked pasta, rice, or cereal; or 1 ounce of cold cereal. Again, starting with breakfast makes it easy.

- **Fish:** A serving of fish—fresh or canned—is about 3 ounces, and you should get 3 servings a week. If you don't eat your weekly allotment, be sure to consume flaxseed or walnuts, because they contain linolenic acid, a precursor to the omega-3 found in fish, which appears to have similar benefits.

- **Legumes:** Get 1–2 servings a day consisting of ¾ cup of cooked beans or 1 tablespoon of peanut butter (despite their name, peanuts are actually legumes— not true members of the nut family).

- **Meat and poultry:** One serving of meat or poultry is 3 ounces. It's okay to have 4 or 5 servings each week of white-meat poultry, but red meat and dark-meat poultry are loaded with artery-clogging saturated fat, and should be eaten only 3 or 4 times a month.

- **Dairy and soy:** Consume 3 servings daily. The serving size is 1 cup of milk, 1 ounce of cheese, or 1 cup of yogurt. Soy foods are improving all the time, so if you haven't liked them in the past, give them another try—you might be surprised. The serving size for these foods is 1 cup of soy milk, 1 cup of soy yogurt, 3 ounces of tofu, or 1 ounce of soy cheese. An egg a day is fine, too.

- **Nuts, seeds, and oils:** 1–2 servings daily are sufficient for this group. Serving sizes are 1 tablespoon of olive or canola oil, 1 tablespoon of nut butter; ⅓ ounce or about 15 nuts, about 20 medium olives, or ⅓ of an avocado.

So here's what a typical day of eating might look like that gives you many of your essential nutrients in roughly 2,000 calories:

Breakfast: 1½ cups raisin-bran cereal with 1 cup nonfat milk and 1 cup blueberries, and 6 ounces calcium-fortified orange juice.

Midmorning Snack: 5 reduced-fat whole-grain crackers with 2 ounces reduced-fat cheddar cheese, and 1 cup green grapes.

Lunch: BLT made with 4 slices turkey bacon, 2 teaspoons fat-free mayonnaise, lettuce, and 3 tomato slices on 2 slices of whole-wheat bread; 1 orange; and 1 low-fat granola bar.

Midafternoon Snack: 1 cup edamame (fresh soy beans), and 1 peach.

Dinner: 5 ounces fish, 2 teaspoons olive oil, 2 ounces polenta, 2 cups greens, and 2 teaspoons pine nuts.

Dessert: 1 banana glazed with 2 teaspoons brown sugar.

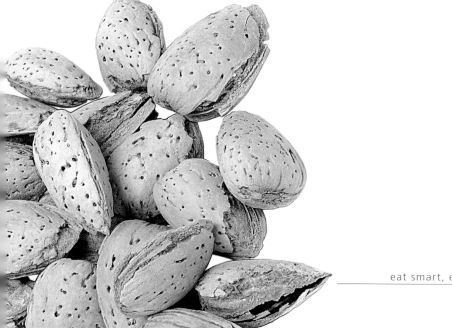

Snacks to Pack

Fiber- and protein-rich nibbles curb hunger pangs and keep you from making choices out of desperation at the vending machine, the cafeteria, or your co-worker's candy bowl. Here are some satisfying picks:

- Reduced-fat sour cream mixed with fresh herbs as a dip for veggies, such as baby carrots.

- Low-fat yogurt topped with dried fruit (such as cranberries, raisins, or apricots) and nuts (such as almonds, peanuts, walnuts, or pistachios).

- Low-fat granola bars with an 8-ounce glass of nonfat milk.

- Baked corn chips with spicy black-bean-and-corn salsa.

- Reduced-fat peanut butter (or any nut butter) on whole-grain bread.

Low-Fat Cooking Equals Good Looking

Selecting wholesome, nutritious foods is the just the first step to creating a healthy, low-fat meal. Certainly the ingredients are part of the process, but the preparation and cooking techniques that you use to turn them into a meal are equally important. So if you love deep-frying, or preparing dinner means peeling back the top of a frozen meal, then it's time for a change.

You don't have to be an accomplished cook to create low-fat cuisine that tastes great. The main challenge to eating well while watching calories is to choose nutrient-dense food and avoid excess dietary fat—without giving up flavor. We'll teach you 5 super-easy, low-fat cooking techniques that you can master in about the time it takes to nuke a Lean Cuisine. Whether you choose to broil, microwave, pressure-cook, steam, or stir-fry, you'll be pleased to know that each method is not only naturally low in fat (requiring little or no oil), but also brings out the zest in foods. We do have one caveat: Because these are quick-cooking techniques, you'll need to ignore that well-known adage and become a cook who *does* watch the pot—in order to help keep it from boiling (or burning or sticking).

Steaming

Steaming is simply cooking food in an enclosed environment infused with steam. You can do this in a variety of ways: with a covered, perforated basket that rests above a pot of boiling water; with wrappings of parchment or foil; with Chinese bamboo steamers that stack on top of a wok; or with convenient electric steamers. This method seals in flavor, eliminating the need for added fats during preparation, and preserves nutrients better than anything except microwaving. It's perfect for fish and shellfish because it doesn't dry out the delicate flesh.

Best Candidates: Vegetables such as asparagus, zucchini, and green beans; pears; chicken breasts, fish fillets, and shellfish. (Halibut, cod, and snapper steam particularly well.)

Equipment: A large pot in which to place collapsible-basket steamers, Chinese-bamboo steamers to stack on top of a wok, or electric steamers. You can also easily create a makeshift version with everyday cooking utensils: Use any deep-frying pan or pot (such as a 6-quart Dutch oven) and place a rack inside, balanced on 2 identical pieces of wood wedged into the bottom. (Make sure the lid is tight fitting.) Spaghetti pots that come with separate smaller baskets that sit up high and fit snugly under the lid are good for this as well.

Cooking Tips: To steam on top of the stove, simply bring water to a boil in your selected vessel, reduce heat so that a strong simmer creates steam, add food to the steaming compartment, cover with a lid, and start the timer. A ¾" to 1" fish fillet takes anywhere from 6–15 minutes to steam, depending upon the fish; vegetables and fruit (such as a bunch of medium-sized asparagus, a pound of green beans, or two cut-up pears) take from 6–10 minutes; a boneless chicken breast clocks in at 20 minutes. Don't bother salting foods, since it just washes off—flavoring is as simple as a twist of lemon upon completion.

Try This: Steam 1 fish fillet by wrapping it in foil with a few garlic cloves, grated fresh ginger, onion, and basil leaves. After squeezing fresh lemon juice over the fish, wrap it up and place it in a steamer basket. Bring 2" of water to a boil in a pot, put the basket over the water, and cover. Steam for about 6 minutes.

Stir-Frying

Cooking at a very high heat for a very short amount of time is the essence of stir-frying. Because food is in the pan so briefly, it should be cut into small, uniform pieces to ensure that every ingredient is cooked thoroughly. This is another method that requires your full attention, as continuous stirring (and sometimes tossing) is necessary to prevent sticking to the pan.

The best way to stir-fry is in a wok, although it's possible to use a large, heavy pan. The sloping sides and rounded bottom are specially designed so food can be quickly browned in the "belly" of the pan and then moved up to the sides, where it finishes cooking more slowly. Traditionally, Chinese woks are made of cast iron and take a while to reach the proper temperature, but most woks today are made of carbon steel, which heats up and cools down more quickly. The wok is placed on a metal ring which sits over the burner; when it's very hot, oil is added, followed by the food.

Best candidates: Broccoli, cabbage, eggplant, bell peppers, mushrooms, pork, chicken, shrimp, scallops, and tofu.

Equipment: A wok or a heavy-gauge skillet.

Cooking tips: Be prepared. Before you begin cooking, vegetables should be properly diced or chopped, meats should be trimmed of fat and sliced, and spices should be laid out on a plate and ready to go. Use extra-virgin olive oil from a spray pump to coat your wok. If you're preparing a meat-and-vegetable dish, brown the meat first, then push it to the sides of the wok before adding the veggies.

Try This: Heat a wok or skillet over high heat, and spray with oil. Add ½ cup chopped onions, 1 minced garlic clove, and a dash of red-pepper flakes; stir-fry for about 30 seconds. Add ½ cup chicken broth and ½ cup white wine; simmer for about 2 minutes. Add ½ pound of medium-size shrimp; cover and cook for 5 minutes.

Broiling

One of the simplest of all cooking methods, broiling cooks by exposing food to direct heat in an electric or gas stove, usually in the bottom drawer of the oven. It gives the same results as grilling, but while a grill heats from below, a broiler cooks from above. Because the heat is constant, all you really need to do is move the food closer to or farther from the flame, depending on how done you want the dish to be. That means that the thinner the cut of food, the closer the heat source should be so that it quickly sears the surface of the food, leaving the interior less done. Because broiling is a dry-heat method (which means no additional oil), lean cuts of beef and chicken work best when marinated first or basted during cooking.

Best Candidates: Salmon, chicken, Cornish game hen, bell peppers, summer squash, zucchini, and onions.

Equipment: Gas or electric stove.

Cooking Tips: Always preheat the broiler for 30 minutes with the rack in place so that foods can be seared quickly. For a ½"-thick piece of meat, allow 6 minutes of cooking time for rare, 9 minutes for medium, and 12 minutes for well-done. For bone-in chicken, allow about 15 minutes per pound. Vegetables take about 10–15 minutes.

Turn all foods halfway through cooking time. To sear (that is, to cook the surface quickly with intense heat), place dish 1" below a preheated broiler for 1–2 minutes per side. For easy cleanup, line your broiler pan with foil.

Try This: For extra flavor, and to keep them from drying out, marinate lean cuts (and even vegetables) for an hour beforehand. Try this marinade with chicken breasts: Combine 3 cloves minced garlic, 1 tablespoon olive oil, the juice and zest of 1 lemon, ¼ cup chopped fresh basil, 1 cup white wine, and salt and pepper to taste.

Microwaving

For all intents and purposes, microwaving is another way of steaming. The foods that do well this way are vegetables, which retain their color along with their nutrients, and fish and chicken, which plump up well compared to beef and pork. There is one thing to look out for, though: Don't use too much water when microwaving veggies, as it can destroy the nutrients. A couple of Tablespoons is enough.

Best Candidates: Beets, broccoli, fish, chicken, potatoes, spinach, carrots, cauliflower, and apples.

Equipment: A medium-size, 750-plus-watt model, with either a carousel to turn the food or a convection system that disperses the waves evenly throughout the oven, will suit most needs. Remember to use microwave-safe glass, ceramic, or plastic cooking vessels. Most glass bowls and baking dishes are okay; ceramic and plastic items will say on the bottom or on the package if they're microwave safe. Never put metal, Styrofoam, or plastic deli containers in the microwave.

Cooking Tips: Cover food to contain the steam and moisture, which keeps food tender and juicy. Although many manuals suggest using plastic wrap as a cover, some studies show that molecules from the wrap can travel into the food. Instead, use covered casserole dishes or a flat, glass plate on top of the container. You can cook two dishes at once by stacking them.

Try This: Flash-cook veggies to retain nutrients. We recommend these tasty options: 6 medium beets, cut up (12 minutes); 2 large sweet potatoes or yams (14 minutes); 1 medium to large head of cauliflower or broccoli, cut into florets (6 minutes); or 2 large bunches of spinach (3 minutes).

Pressure-Cooking

Food cooked in a pressure cooker requires very little water and time, which means that vitamins and minerals are kept intact. This device seals in steam created by boiling liquid, which intensifies flavors, meaning that you won't need to add any oil or fat for taste or richness. In fact, you barely need to season the food at all. Soups and stews that would usually take hours to simmer on the stove or a whole chicken can be ready in 15 minutes, rice in 5, and most vegetables in about 3.

Best Candidates: Artichokes, potatoes, beans, beef, chicken, lamb, risotto, soups, and stews.

Equipment: There are three types of pressure cookers: the old-fashioned "jiggler" or weight-valve, the developed weight-valve, and the spring-valve. The valve on each model serves as a pressure regulator and tells you when it's time to adjust the heat. (They all feature safety valves as well, which allow excess pressure to escape; and most have safety locks that make them impossible to open until the pressure has fully dropped.) The spring-valve is the most precise and easiest for beginners to use.

Cooking Tips: Use a timer when pressure-cooking. This method works so quickly that every second really counts. Don't fill your cooker more than ⅔ full, and when cooking foods that expand (such as beans or rice), only fill it halfway to allow for the buildup of steam and pressure.

Try This: Beef Stew with Orange and Rosemary: In a 5-quart pressure cooker, heat 1 tablespoon olive oil on high heat. Add 1½ pounds lean beef cut into 1" cubes, and cook until well browned on all sides. Remove and set aside.

Reduce heat and add 1 chopped onion, 1 clove garlic, and 2 Tablespoons beef broth. Cook about 1 minute. Add ½ cup more of beef broth, ½ cup dry red wine, 2 Tablespoons tomato paste, ½ teaspoon dried rosemary leaves, 1 teaspoon finely grated orange peel, 1 teaspoon dried thyme, 1 bay leaf, and black pepper to taste. Stir well to dissolve tomato paste, then add beef. Close lid and bring pressure to high. Reduce heat as needed, and cook for 15 minutes.

Weight-Loss-Friendly Gadgets

Having these items on hand will make it easy to decrease the amount of unhealthful fat in your food while adding flavor and variety.

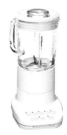

- **Blender:** for making low-fat marinades, salad dressing, sauces, dips, smoothies, shakes, and pureed desserts. Good choices are the KitchenAid 5-Speed Ultra Power Blender and the Cuisinart SmartPower Basics 18-Speed Electronic Blender.

- **Grinder:** for grinding your own coffee to make fresh skim-milk lattes and mocha drinks; also great for grinding spices (to add fat-free flavor when cooking) and nuts (for homemade nut butters). A good choice is the Krups Coffee and Spice Grinder.

- **Vegetable Cutter:** makes it easier to add fruits and vegetables to your meals by quickly chopping them into uniform pieces. A good choice is the Transparent Rapid Food Chopper by Zyliss.

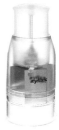

- **Oil Sprayer:** a measured amount of your favorite oil (such as an herb-infused olive oil) goes perfectly on salads or in cooking when it comes from a pump sprayer. Good choices are the Cuisipro SprayPump and Misto Gourmet Olive Oil Sprayer.

You can find these and other such useful gadgets at **www. cooking.com**, **tabletools.com**, and **surlatable.com**.

Food as Fuel

Now that you're committed to working out regularly, you might have some specific nutrition needs over and above general good eating. For instance, what if you're logging miles on the treadmill, when suddenly you "bonk"—you feel weak, tired, and completely drained of energy? The culprit could very well be your diet.

According to Lona Sandon, R.D., an assistant professor of clinical nutrition at the University of Texas Southwestern Medical Center at Dallas and a spokeswoman for the American Dietetic Association (ADA), people trying to get in shape and/or lose weight are among those most likely to consume too few calories. That has a powerful effect on your energy level, but eating too much also can leave you feeling sluggish. Essentially, you need to eat the right amount of calories—and the right kinds at the appropriate times—if you want to function at full throttle. Here's how to fuel yourself most effectively, and stop the slumps:

1. Get the balance right. When it comes to optimizing your energy level, not all calories are created equal. "The source of the calories makes a difference," confirms Susan Bowerman, M.S., R.D., assistant director of the Center for Human Nutrition at the University of California, Los Angeles. "Get a good balance of nutrients. Carbohydrates are the primary fuel your body uses, and protein, which often has fat in it naturally, keeps you feeling full and satisfied."

She recommends consuming at least half of each day's total calories from carbohydrates, especially high-fiber sources such as fruits, vegetables, and whole grains; up to 30 percent from protein; and around 20 percent from fat.

Carbohydrates are digested faster than the two other macro-nutrients, protein and fat, so they provide quick energy. But if you carbo-load on a supersized fat-free muffin at breakfast, you may crash before lunch because you didn't get any protein or fat, which yield longer-term energy that sustains you between meals. Do keep in mind that a little fat goes a long way, however, providing nine calories per gram, versus four calories per gram for carbohydrates or protein. Bowerman notes that you generally don't need to add fat to your diet, but if you do, the best sources are nuts, avocados, and olive oil.

You might find this advice confusing because everyone seems to be touting a high-protein diet, claiming that carbs are detrimental to your weight and your health. But we know better: You need carbohydrates for key bodily functions. In addition to providing fuel for your muscles, they also help your brain function properly, control your appetite, maintain even blood-sugar levels, and help promote weight loss. Complex, high-fiber sources produce a slower rise in blood sugar than simple carbs do, which means that they give you time-released energy and prevent those peaks and valleys in your blood sugar that can cause cravings and poor food choices.

2. Eat at the right times. Aim for three similarly sized meals and two small snacks a day, spaced three or four hours apart, and try to incorporate some of each macronutrient at every meal. This will provide you with a steady supply of energy to keep you going strong all day and will prevent you from getting so hungry that you overeat at your next meal.

3. Eat enough. Not sure if you're consuming too few or too many calories? You can calculate your needs with the widely used Harris-Benedict formula in Your Daily-Calorie Needs (page 346). If you don't want to do that much math, Sandon offers this simple calculation: If you're sedentary, multiply your weight in pounds by 13; if you exercise moderately (about three or four times a week), multiply your weight by 15; and if you're very active (exercising an hour nearly every day), multiply your weight by 20. Just note that these formulas don't take lean body mass into account, so they aren't always accurate for women with a lot of muscle or a high body-fat percentage.

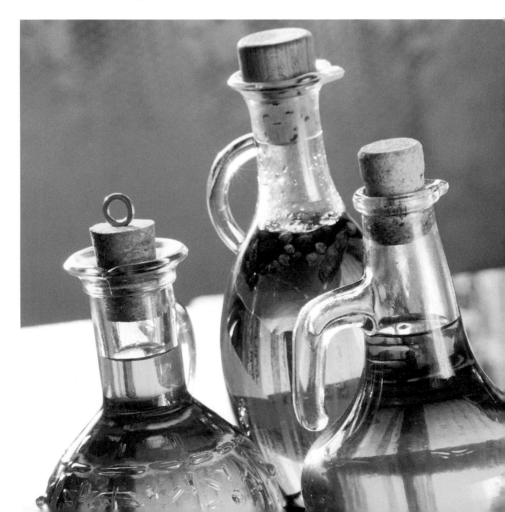

Your Daily-Calorie Needs

1. **Determine your Resting Metabolic Rate (RMR)**
    Calculate your weight
    in kilograms by dividing
    your weight in pounds by 2.2   _____

    Calculate your height
    in centimeters by multiplying
    your height in inches by 2.54   _____

    Multiply your weight
    in kilograms by 9.6 and add 655   _____

    Multiply your height
    in centimeters by 1.8 and
    add it to the above number   _____

    Multiply your age
    by 4.7 and subtract it from the
    above number to get your RMR   _____

2. **Factor in your daily activity**
    Multiply your RMR by the appropriate
    activity factor. If you are:

    Sedentary (little or no activity):
    RMR x 1.2   _____

    Slightly active (light exercise/sports
    1–3 days a week): RMR x 1.375   _____

    Moderately active (moderate exercise/
    sports 3–5 days a week): RMR x 1.55   _____

Very active (strenuous exercise/sports
6–7 days a week): RMR x 1.725   _____

Extra active (very strenuous exercise
twice a day or a physical job): RMR x 1.9   _____

Result: Your final figure represents the minimum number of
daily calories needed to maintain your current weight.

4. Drink up. It's important to stay well hydrated, so be sure to drink at least six 8-ounce glasses of water daily. (Bowerman notes that decaffeinated tea and coffee, as well as soup, also count toward meeting fluid needs.)

5. Choose vitamin-rich foods. Specific vitamins and minerals also help keep us energized. For example, iron deficiency, which leads to anemia, can be a cause of fatigue in women. Good dietary sources of iron include dark-green leafy vegetables, fortified cereals, and red meat. Other causes of anemia are a lack of folic acid (found in leafy greens; citrus fruits and juices; legumes; nuts; and fortified foods, including some cereals, breads, and pastas) or not enough vitamin B$_{12}$ (abundant in eggs, red meat, fish, and milk). If you suspect that you may be anemic, ask your doctor for a blood test.

Another mineral helpful for fighting fatigue is magnesium (found in nuts, spinach, and legumes), which helps the body use energy from food.

Q. If I want lose 15 pounds, which should I keep track of: carbs, calories, or fat grams?

A. Count calories. It's your most useful weight-loss tool, although it's not something you need to do forever, counsels Boston nutritional consultant Heidi Reichenberger, M.S., R.D., a spokeswoman for the American Dietetic Association. "The bottom line is, the number of calories you eat will determine whether you lose weight, gain weight, or stay the same," she explains.

There's no reason to track fat grams, though. Even when you reduce your fat intake, it's still possible to consume way too many calories. For instance, a 44-ounce 7-Eleven Super Big Gulp cola contains no fat, but has nearly 600 calories!

And despite the popularity of low-carb diets, there's no benefit to counting carbohydrates, either. "There aren't many carbs in fried chicken or a greasy cheeseburger, but you could easily go way overboard on calories," Reichenberger points out.

If you have no idea how many calories you're averaging a day—and most people don't—it can be an eye-opening experience to keep track for a week. Write down everything that you eat and drink, plus the amounts, and use food labels and the U.S. Department of Agriculture's Nutrient Database (**www.nal.usda.gov/fnic/cgi-bin/nut_search.pl**) to estimate your daily-calorie intake. Then look for easy ways to cut back here and there, such as choosing a latte made with nonfat milk instead of whole milk (savings: 100 calories).

If you follow our guidelines, watch your portion sizes, and eat a wide variety of foods, you shouldn't have to track anything too closely. "That just takes the fun out of eating," says Reichenberger.

Getting Your Fill

Following the "eating for extra oomph" rules might seem complicated—until you look at some sample meal plans. Keep yourself going strong by mixing and matching these menu ideas for three meals and two snacks according to your calorie needs. If it's been several hours since you last ate, have one of your snacks about an hour before exercising (don't forget that carbs fuel working muscles). As you become familiar with ingredients and serving sizes, you'll start concocting your own favorites.

Breakfast

- 1 whole-grain English muffin with 1 tablespoon peanut butter and 1 sliced banana (355 calories)

- 2 eggs scrambled with ½ cup spinach leaves, and 2 slices whole-grain toast with 2 teaspoons all-fruit preserves (311 calories)

- 1 cup raisin bran or high-fiber, whole-grain cereal with ½ cup low-fat yogurt or calcium-fortified, low-fat soy milk; topped with ½ cup berries (strawberries, blueberries, or blackberries) (320 calories)

Lunch

- 4 ounces ground turkey breast, sautéed and spooned into 2 whole-wheat tortillas; top each with ¼ cup each chopped lettuce, low-fat shredded cheddar cheese, and prepared salsa (363 calories)

- 1 whole-wheat pita pocket stuffed with 2 tablespoons prepared hummus; ⅓ cup each shredded red cabbage and sliced zucchini; 1 sliced tomato; and 3 ounces shredded, cooked chicken breast (416 calories)

- 2 cups prepared lentil soup and a side salad made with 2 cups chopped romaine lettuce; ¼ cup each diced cucumbers, red bell pepper, and carrots; and 1 tablespoon balsamic vinegar mixed with 1 teaspoon olive oil (337 calories)

Dinner

- 5 ounces grilled fish (salmon, tuna, trout, or tilapia) with 8 asparagus spears and 1 cup wild rice (450 calories)

- 2 cups mixed-lettuce greens topped with 4 ounces cooked lean-beef-tenderloin strips; 1 cup diced, cooked red potatoes; and ½ cup corn; topped with 2 tablespoons low-fat ranch dressing (462 calories)

- 2 cups prepared vegetarian chili with a 2-ounce whole-grain roll (486 calories)

Snacks

- 1 cup fresh broccoli florets or 12 baby carrots dunked in ¼ cup low-fat, plain yogurt mixed with 2 teaspoons chopped fresh dill (with broccoli: 61 calories; with carrots: 82 calories)

- 6 whole-grain crackers with 2 tablespoons prepared hummus (113 calories)

- ¼ cup mixed nuts (214 calories)

Pre-workout Snacks

- 1 cup low-fat (1 percent) cottage cheese with ½ cup cubed cantaloupe (192 calories)

- 6 whole-grain crackers with ½ cup sliced, raw zucchini and 1 ounce cheddar cheese (184 calories)

- Smoothie made from 1 cup nonfat milk blended with ½ cup berries (strawberries, raspberries, blackberries, or a mixture) (116 calories)

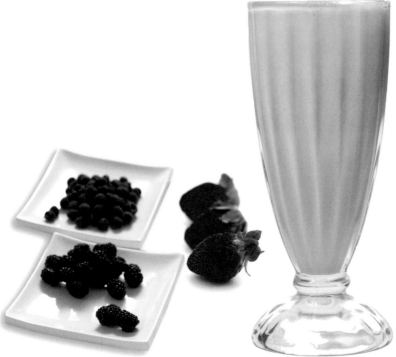

Misstep:

Crash dieting, because deprivation doesn't do you any good. For starters, a dramatic reduction in calories often has a diuretic effect, says Sue Cummings, clinical-program coordinator at Massachusetts General Hospital Weight Center in Boston. That means that the initial drop you see on the scale isn't fat melting away; it's simply water loss. If you eat less than 1,200 calories a day—the minimum amount most women need to keep all systems go—then you'll likely burn lean-muscle mass instead of fat, confirms Lona Sandon, R.D., and American Dietetic Association spokesperson. And if you drop below the minimum needed just for breathing and organ function (this amount varies, but is typically around 900 calories daily), your body shifts into starvation mode. In this state, it won't want to give up a bit of its precious energy stores (that is, fat), Other crash-diet drawbacks include low energy, disrupted sleep, hunger, and extreme irritability.

Post-Makeover Meals

Now that you know how to stock your cabinets and fridge for easier weight loss, how much to eat daily, and how to cook, you'll need some simple, yet delicious, recipes that comply with our guidelines for healthful eating. But you don't have to be a slave to your newly made-over kitchen: Prepare large enough quantities to freeze so that you'll always have a hearty, healthful meal available to eat in minutes.

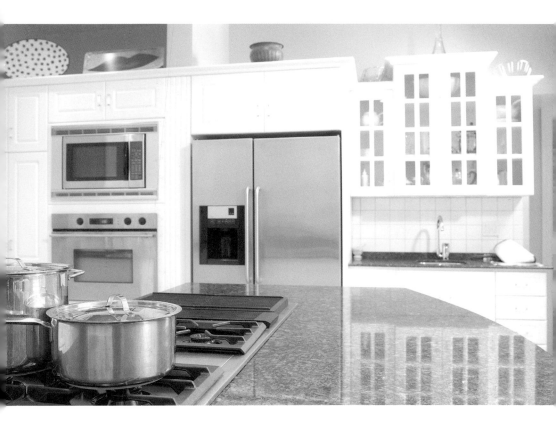

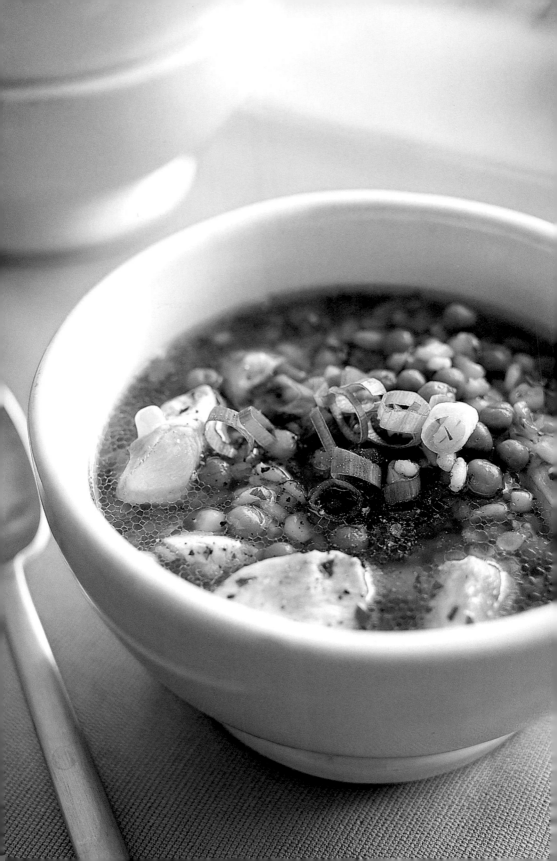

Chicken-Barley Soup with Vegetables

Serves 4
Prep time: 5 minutes
Cook time: 15 minutes

2 teaspoons olive oil
4 green onions, chopped, with white and green parts divided
1 pound skinless, boneless chicken breast, cut into ½" pieces
1 teaspoon dried thyme
2 bay leaves
Three 14.5-ounce cans reduced-sodium chicken broth
⅔ cup quick-cooking barley
½ cup frozen peas
1 tablespoon chopped fresh parsley
Salt and ground-black pepper

Heat oil in a large saucepan over medium-high heat. Add white parts of onions and cook 1 minute. Add chicken and cook until browned on all sides (about 3 minutes), stirring frequently. Toss in thyme and bay leaves; stir to coat chicken and onions.

Add broth and barley and bring to a boil. Reduce heat to low; cover and simmer 10 minutes or until tender. Stir in corn and peas and simmer 1 minute longer. Remove from heat and add parsley. Season with salt and pepper to taste. Remove bay leaves and serve topped with green parts of onions.

Nutrition score per serving (1½ cups): 296 calories, 18% fat (6 g; 1 g sat.), 36% carbs (27 g), 46% protein (34 g), 28 mg calcium, 2 mg iron, 4 g fiber, 692 mg sodium.

Egg Strata

Serves 4
Prep time: 10 minutes
Cook time: 6–10 minutes

Nonstick cooking spray
8 slices whole-grain pumpernickel bread, cut into ½" cubes
One 14.5-ounce can diced tomatoes with basil, garlic,
    and oregano (such as Hunt's)
1 cup shredded, reduced-fat cheddar cheese
1 cup nonfat milk
4 large eggs
2 teaspoons Dijon mustard
¼ teaspoon ground-black pepper
2 Tablespoons grated Parmesan cheese

Preheat broiler. Coat a microwave-safe shallow baking dish (about 7" x 11") with cooking spray. Arrange pumpernickel cubes in the bottom of dish. Spoon tomatoes over bread, then sprinkle cheddar cheese over tomatoes. Set aside.

In a small bowl, whisk together milk, eggs, Dijon mustard, and black pepper. Pour mixture over tomato- and cheese-topped bread; then sprinkle with Parmesan. Cover dish with fitted lid or paper towel. Microwave on high 6–10 minutes (it's best to undercook, so check frequently) until eggs are set, rotating dish once during cooking. Place under broiler for 1 minute, or until top is golden brown. Let stand 2 minutes before slicing into 4 equal portions.

Nutrition score per serving (¼ of strata): 373 calories, 31% fat (13 g; 6 g sat.), 42% carbs (39 g), 27% protein (25 g), 435 mg calcium, 3 mg iron, 6 g fiber, 1,013 mg sodium.

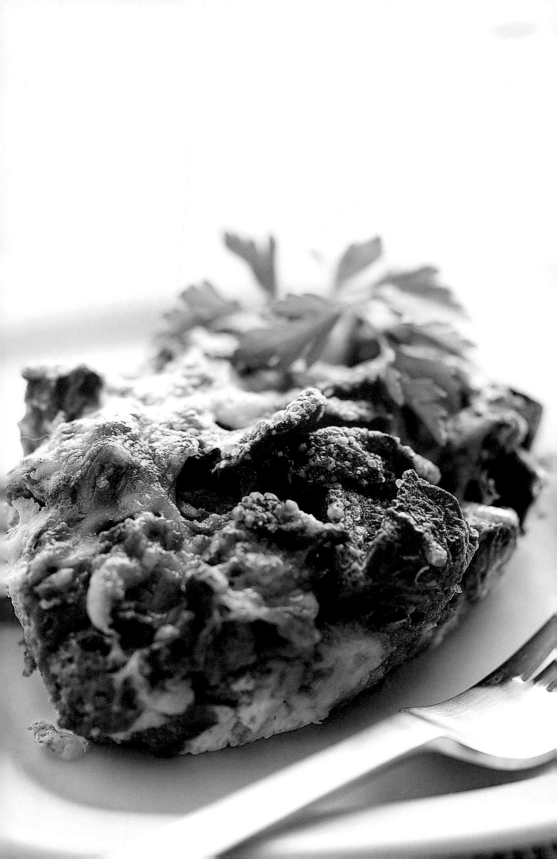

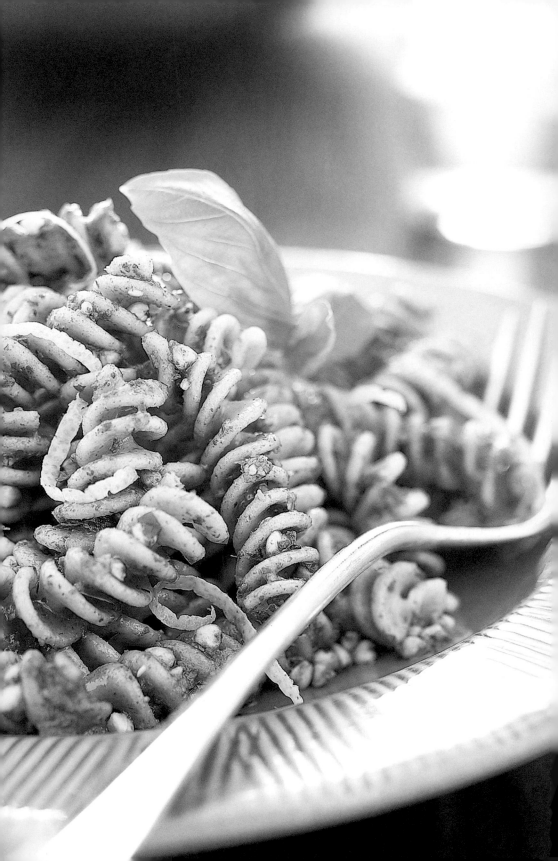

Kasha and Pasta with Lemon Pesto

Serves 2
Prep time: 5 minutes
Cook time: 10–12 minutes

4 ounces whole-wheat pasta spirals (or other shape)
3 tablespoons medium-granulation kasha (roasted buckwheat)
1 egg white (or 2 tablespoons refrigerated egg whites)
Nonstick cooking spray
½ cup fat-free chicken broth
¼ teaspoon salt
¼ teaspoon ground-black pepper
¼ cup prepared pesto (such as Buitoni)
3 tablespoons fresh lemon juice

Cook pasta according to package directions. Drain and cover with foil; set aside.

Meanwhile, in a small bowl, combine kasha and egg white, stirring to coat kasha. Spray a small saucepan with cooking spray and set pan over medium heat. Add kasha and cook 2–3 minutes, until egg is cooked and kasha kernels separate. Add broth, salt, and pepper; cover and simmer 7 minutes, until liquid is absorbed. Add kasha to pasta and stir.

Whisk together pesto and lemon juice. Pour mixture over pasta and stir to coat. Serve warm or at room temperature.

Nutrition score per serving (1¼ cups): 433 calories, 31% fat (15 g; 3 g sat.), 55% carbs (59.5 g), 14% protein (15 g), 103 mg calcium, 2 mg iron, 6 g fiber, 458 mg sodium.

Pressed-Tofu Kebabs, Thai Style

Serves 4
Prep time: 20 minutes (plus 60 minutes to press tofu)
Cook time: 5–8 minutes

One 15-ounce container firm or extra-firm tofu
¼ cup fresh lime juice
1 tablespoon chopped, fresh cilantro
2 teaspoons reduced-sodium soy sauce
2 teaspoons peanut oil
1 clove garlic, minced
⅛ teaspoon ground-black pepper
1 red bell pepper, cut into 1" cubes
4 green onions, cut crosswise
1 cup whole-wheat couscous, cooked according
    to package directions without added fat
½ cup prepared Thai-peanut sauce

Wrap the tofu in a clean cotton kitchen towel, place it in a shallow pan (to collect any water), and then top the tofu with a heavy cutting board. Put pots on top of the cutting board (to weigh it down). Let the tofu stand for 30–60 minutes, depending on how firm you like it; drain the pan halfway through pressing, if necessary.

In a shallow dish, whisk together lime juice, cilantro, soy sauce, peanut oil, garlic, and black pepper. Add pressed tofu and turn to coat. Cover with plastic and marinate 15 minutes (or up to 24 hours, refrigerated).

Preheat grill or broiler.

Remove tofu from marinade (reserve marinade) and cut the tofu into 16 pieces. Alternate pieces of tofu, red pepper, and green onion on wooden skewers; brush with marinade. Grill or broil 5–8 minutes, until vegetables are charred and tofu is hot, turning frequently and brushing with marinade halfway through cooking. Serve kebabs with couscous, with the peanut sauce on the side for dipping.

Nutrition score per serving (2 kebabs, ½ cup couscous, and 2 Tablespoons peanut sauce): 370 calories, 22% fat (9 g; <1 g sat.), 57% carbs (53 g), 21% protein (19 g), 68 mg calcium, 3 mg iron, 9 g fiber, 746 mg sodium.

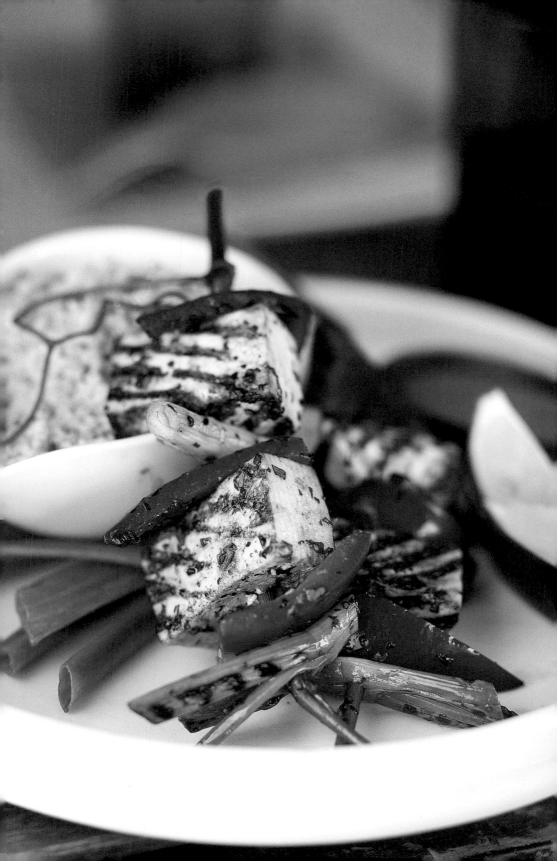

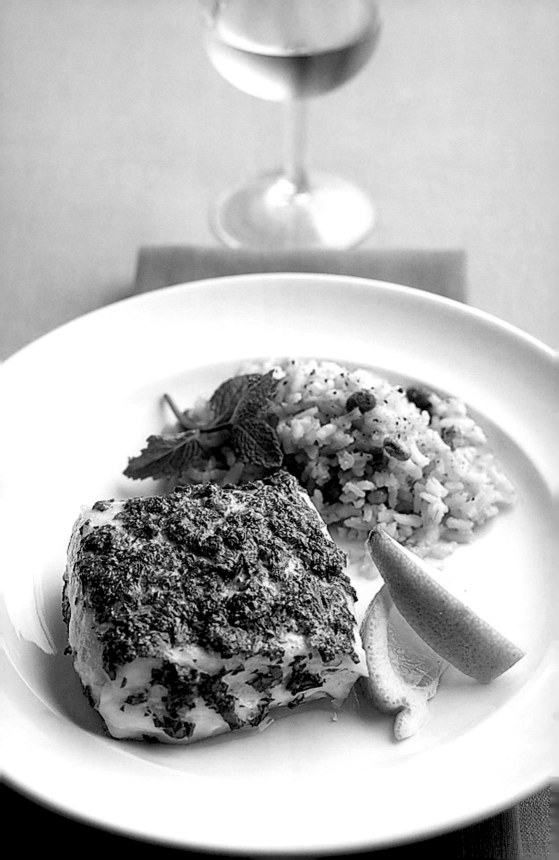

Herb-Crusted Halibut with Rice Pilaf

Serves 4
Prep time: 10 minutes
Cook time: 18 minutes

Nonstick cooking spray
Salt and ground-black pepper
Four 5-ounce halibut fillets, about 1" thick
    (or other fish such as trout, cod, or tilapia)
2 tablespoons chopped fresh basil
2 tablespoons chopped fresh mint
½ teaspoon dried mustard
3 tablespoons olive oil, divided
2 shallots, minced
2 cloves garlic, minced
1 cup instant brown rice
1¼ cups reduced-sodium chicken or vegetable broth, or water
¼ cup roasted soybeans

Preheat oven to 425° F. Coat a large baking sheet with cooking spray.

Salt and pepper both sides of fish to taste. In a small bowl, combine basil, mint, mustard, and 1 teaspoon of oil. Mix well and rub over both sides of fish. Transfer fish to prepared baking sheet and roast for 10–12 minutes, until fork-tender (no need to turn the fish).

Meanwhile, heat remaining oil in a saucepan over medium-high heat. Add shallots and garlic and cook 1 minute; add rice and cook 1 minute more. Add broth and bring mixture to a boil. Reduce heat to low, cover, and simmer 10 minutes. Remove from heat, add soybeans, and fluff with a fork. Serve rice pilaf alongside roasted fish.

Nutrition score per serving (1 halibut filet, ⅔ cup of pilaf): 272 calories, 28% fat (8 g; 1 g sat.), 30% carbs (20 g), 42% protein (29 g), 68 mg calcium, 1 mg iron, 1 g fiber, 341 mg sodium.

Shrimp Fra Diavolo

Serves 4
Prep time: 10 minutes
Cook time: 18 minutes

2 teaspoons olive oil
4 cloves garlic, minced
One 28-ounce can diced tomatoes
1 teaspoon dried oregano
½ teaspoon crushed-red-pepper flakes (or more to taste)
1 pound medium shrimp, peeled and deveined (24–30 shrimp) or
    1 pound cleaned, frozen shrimp (thawed)
¼ cup chopped fresh basil
12 ounces whole-wheat linguine

Heat olive oil in a large saucepan over medium-high heat. Add minced garlic and cook 1 minute. Add tomatoes, oregano, and red-pepper flakes and bring to a boil. Reduce heat to low, cover, and simmer 15 minutes.

Meanwhile, cook linguine according to package direction. Drain and set aside.

Add shrimp to simmering tomato sauce and cook 2 minutes, until bright pink and cooked through. Remove from heat and stir in basil.

Transfer linguine to individual plates, top with tomato-shrimp mixture, and serve.

Nutrition score per serving (1½ cups): 448 calories, 9% fat (4 g; 1 g sat.), 64% carbs (72 g), 27% protein (30 g), 84 mg calcium, 6 mg iron, 11 g fiber, 596 mg sodium.

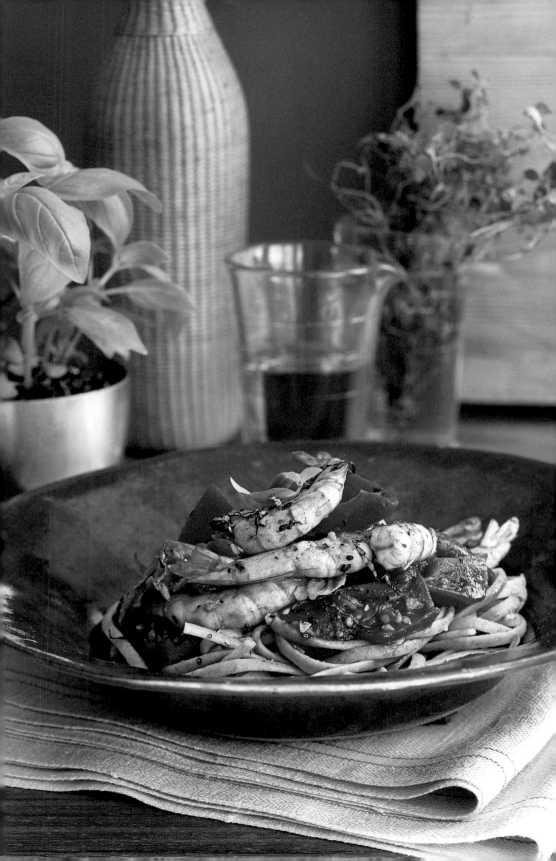

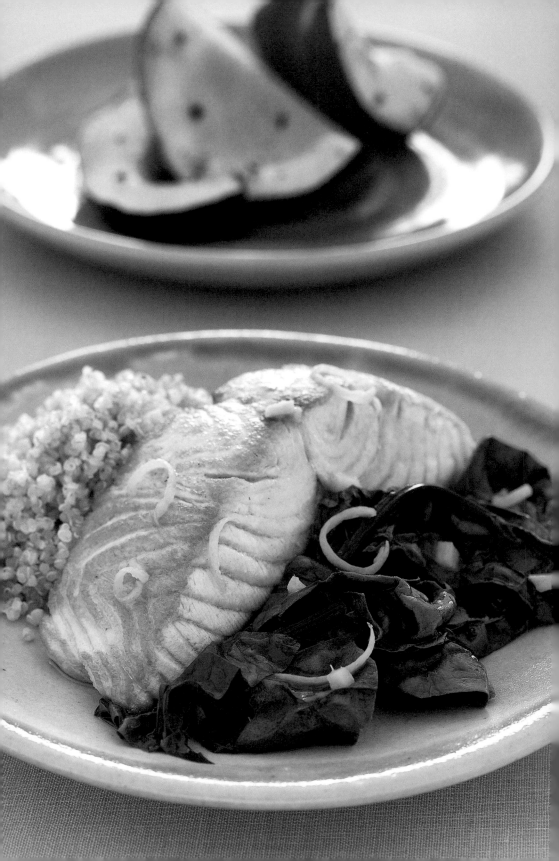

Gingered Salmon
with Quinoa and Swiss Chard

Serves 2
Prep time: 5 minutes
Cook time: 10–12 minutes

½ cup uncooked quinoa
½ cup vegetable broth
2 teaspoons minced fresh ginger
2 teaspoons fresh lemon juice
1 teaspoon finely grated lemon zest
1 teaspoon cornstarch
Nonstick cooking spray
One 6-ounce salmon fillet, about 1" thick
Salt and ground-black pepper
2 cups chopped fresh Swiss chard, rinsed well

Combine quinoa and 1 cup water in small saucepan and set over medium-high heat. Bring to a boil, reduce heat to low, cover, and simmer 10–12 minutes, until liquid is absorbed. Fluff with a fork and season to taste.

Meanwhile, in a small bowl, whisk together broth, ginger, lemon juice, lemon zest, and cornstarch; set aside.

Coat a large nonstick skillet with cooking spray and set pan over medium-high heat. Season both sides of salmon with salt and pepper and place in the pan, skin side up. Cook 2 minutes; flip and cook 2 more minutes. Add broth mixture and simmer 30 seconds. Arrange Swiss chard around salmon, cover pan, and cook 1 minute, until greens are wilted and salmon is cooked through. Serve half of the salmon and Swiss chard with half of the quinoa on the side.

Nutrition score per serving (3 ounces salmon, ½ cup Swiss chard, ½ cup quinoa): 306 calories, 26% fat (9 g; 1 g sat.), 36% carbs (27.5 g), 38% protein (29 g), 62 mg calcium, 1 mg iron, 3 g fiber, 248 mg sodium.

King Mackerel (or Trout) Enchiladas

Serves 2
Prep time: 10 minutes
Cook time: 20 minutes

One 8-ounce king mackerel or trout fillet,
    skinned and cut into ½" cubes
2 tablespoons fat-free Italian dressing (vinaigrette style)
1 tablespoon all-purpose flour
Nonstick cooking spray
½ cup onion, minced
1 green bell pepper, minced
1 cup prepared salsa (divided use)
¼ cup chopped fresh cilantro
Two 8" whole-wheat tortillas
¼ cup shredded reduced-fat Mexican cheese blend (Sargento)
    or reduced-fat cheddar cheese

Combine king mackerel or trout cubes and fat-free Italian dressing in a shallow dish and stir to coat fish with dressing. Let stand 15 minutes; then add flour and toss to coat.

Preheat oven to 350° F. Coat a baking dish with cooking spray and set aside.

Spray a large nonstick skillet with cooking spray and set pan over medium-high heat. Add onion and green pepper and sauté 2 minutes, until soft. Add king mackerel or trout and cook 2 minutes, until fish is opaque, stirring constantly. Stir in the cilantro and ½ cup of the salsa and mix well. Remove from heat.

Spoon fish mixture onto whole-wheat tortillas, roll up, and place seam side down in prepared baking dish. Spoon remaining salsa over top and sprinkle with shredded cheese.

Bake uncovered for 20 minutes, until cheese melts.

Nutrition score per serving (1 enchilada): 445 calories, 40% fat (20 g; 5 g sat.), 28% carbs (31 g), 32% protein (34 g), 176 mg calcium, 2 mg iron, 15 g fiber, 1,918 mg sodium.

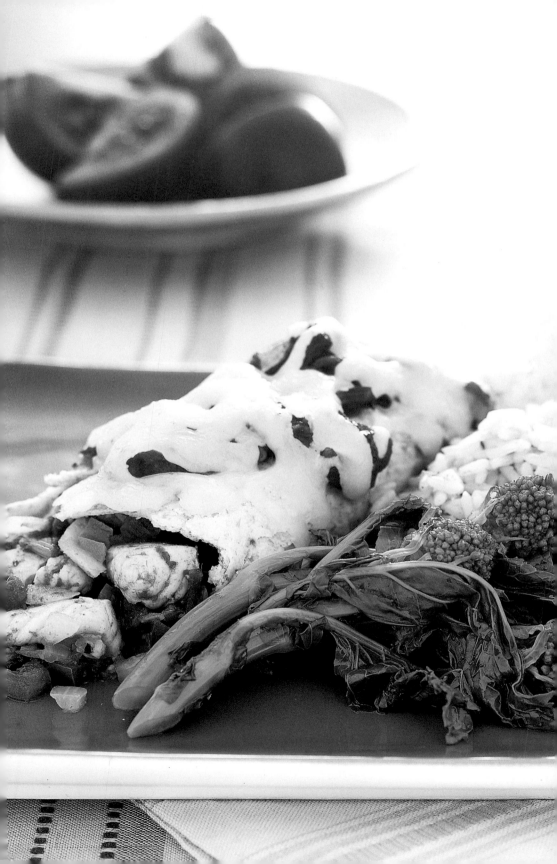

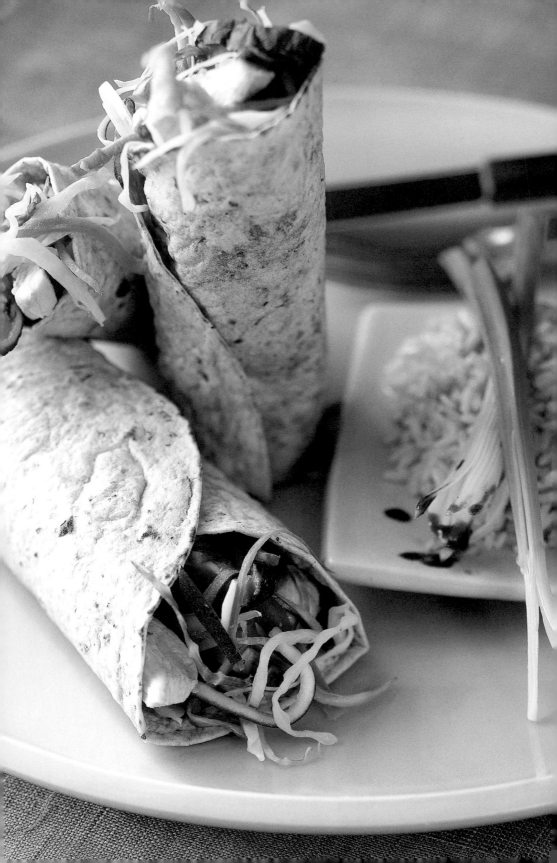

Stir-Fry Mu Shu Vegetables with Chicken

Serves 4
Prep time: 20 minutes
Cook time: 5–6 minutes

4 dried black-Chinese mushrooms or dried shiitake mushrooms
⅓ cup fat-free chicken or vegetable broth
1 tablespoon reduced-sodium soy sauce
2 teaspoons cornstarch
2 teaspoons sesame oil
2 cloves garlic, minced
1 tablespoon fresh ginger root, minced
1 pound skinless, boneless chicken breasts,
    cut into ¼"-thick strips
4 cups shredded green cabbage or packaged coleslaw mix
1 carrot, cut into matchstick-size pieces
1 small zucchini, cut into matchstick-size pieces
2 green onions, sliced diagonally into ¼" pieces
Eight 6" whole-wheat or spinach tortillas
¼ cup hoisin sauce

Soak dried mushrooms in ½ cup warm water for 20 minutes. Drain, reserving mushroom liquid; remove and discard any stems and thinly sliced caps.

Whisk together broth, soy sauce, and cornstarch; set aside.

Heat oil in wok or large skillet over high heat. Add minced garlic and ginger and stir-fry for 30 seconds. Add chicken and stir-fry for 2–3 minutes, until no longer pink. Add cabbage, carrots, zucchini, green onions, reserved mushrooms, and mushroom liquid and stir-fry for 1 minute, until cabbage wilts. Add cornstarch mixture and simmer 1 minute, until liquid thickens. Remove from heat.

Wrap tortillas in plastic and heat in the microwave for 15 seconds to soften. Spoon 1½ teaspoons of hoisin sauce on each tortilla, add chicken and vegetable mixture, and roll up.

Nutrition score per serving (2 tortillas, 1 cup chicken-and-vegetable filling): 390 calories, 14% fat (6 g; 1 g sat.), 50% carbs (49 g), 36% protein (35 g), 102 mg calcium, 2 mg iron, 23 g fiber, 927 mg sodium.

Olive-Crusted
Chicken with Quinoa and Vegetables

Serves 4
Prep time: 10 minutes
Cook time: 25 minutes

Nonstick cooking spray
½ cup pitted kalamata olives
¼ cup green olives (stuffed with pimento)
1 tablespoon capers, drained
1 clove garlic, chopped
Four 4-ounce skinless, boneless chicken
    breast halves, rinsed and patted dry
1 cup uncooked quinoa
2 carrots, peeled and diced
½ cup frozen green peas (thawed)
⅓ cup minced red onion
2 tablespoons chopped fresh basil
1½ tablespoons red-wine vinegar
2 teaspoons olive oil
Salt and ground-black pepper

Preheat oven to 400° F. Coat a large baking sheet with cooking spray.

To make the olive crust: In a food processor, combine olives, capers, and garlic. Process until smooth.

Place chicken on prepared baking sheet and coat the top with the olive mixture. Bake 25 minutes, until cooked through.

Meanwhile, make the quinoa salad: Rinse quinoa under cool, running water and drain. Combine quinoa and 2 cups of water in a medium saucepan; set the pan over high heat and bring to a boil. Reduce heat to low, cover, and cook 10 minutes, until liquid is absorbed and quinoa is translucent. Remove from heat and stir in carrots, peas, onion, basil, vinegar, and oil. Season with salt and black pepper to taste, and serve alongside chicken.

Nutrition score per serving (1 chicken breast, ⅔ cup quinoa salad): 402 calories, 28% fat (12 g; 1.6 g sat.), 39% carbs (39 g), 33% protein (33 g), 63 mg calcium, 6 mg iron, 5 g fiber, 580 mg sodium.

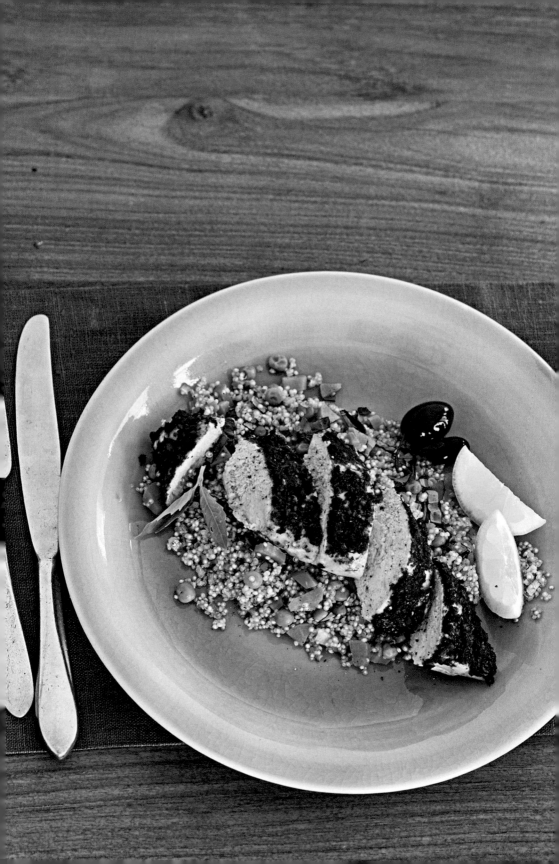

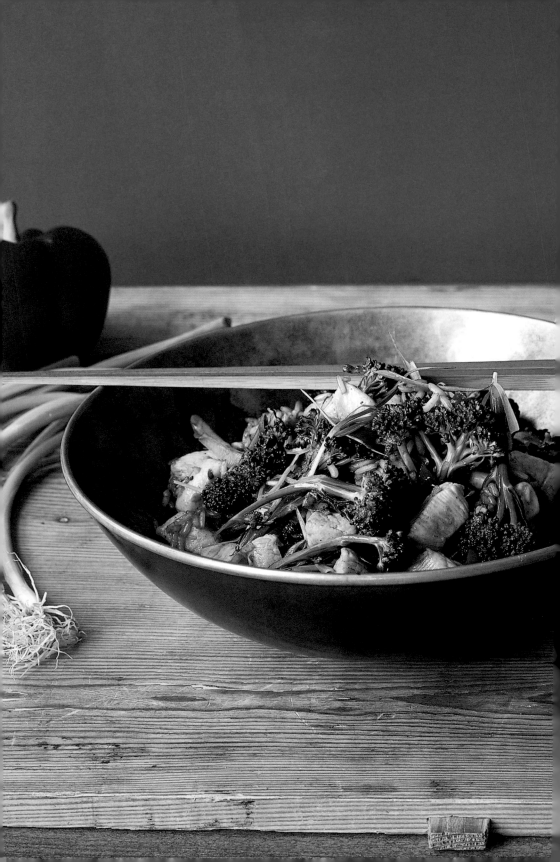

Sesame Fried Rice with Chicken

Serves 4
Prep time: 10 minutes
Cook time: 30 minutes

2 teaspoons dark-sesame oil
2 cloves garlic, minced
1 pound skinless, boneless chicken breasts, cut into 1" pieces
1 cup uncooked brown rice
1 tablespoon reduced-sodium soy sauce
2 cups reduced-sodium chicken broth or water
¼ teaspoon salt
2 cups broccoli florets
1 red bell pepper, seeded and diced
¼ cup chopped green onions

Heat oil in a medium saucepan over medium heat. Add garlic and sauté 1 minute. Add chicken and sauté 3–5 minutes, until golden on all sides, stirring frequently. Add rice and cook 1 minute; then add soy sauce and stir to coat. Add chicken broth, salt, and pepper and bring mixture to a boil. Reduce heat, cover, and simmer 20 minutes.

Arrange broccoli and red pepper on top of rice, cover, and cook 5 more minutes, until vegetables are crisp and tender and liquid is absorbed. Stir vegetables into rice. Remove from heat, stir in green onions, and serve.

Nutrition score per serving (1 cup): 299 calories, 19% fat (6 g; 1 g sat.), 37% carbs (28 g), 44% protein (33 g), 53 mg calcium, 2 mg iron, 4 g fiber, 576 mg sodium.

Meatballs with Mushroom Sauce Over Smashed Sweet Potatoes

Serves 4
Prep time: 20 minutes
Cook time: 12 minutes

1 pound sweet potatoes (2 large), peeled and cut into 2" cubes
4 teaspoons olive oil (divided use)
½ teaspoon ground-black pepper (divided use)
1 pound extra-lean ground sirloin (about 90–95% lean)
½ cup diced onion
¼ cup seasoned bread crumbs
2 egg whites
2 tablespoons chopped fresh parsley
1 cup sliced fresh shiitake or other wild mushrooms
1 teaspoon dried thyme
1 cup reduced-sodium beef broth
1 tablespoon cornstarch
¼ cup sherry

To make the smashed potatoes, place sweet potatoes in a large saucepan and add enough water to cover. Set pan over high heat and bring to a boil. Cook 8 minutes, until fork-tender. Drain and transfer to a large bowl. Add 2 teaspoons of the olive oil, ¼ teaspoon of the salt, and ¼ teaspoon of the pepper and smash together with a fork until mixture is lumpy.

Meanwhile, to make the meatballs, combine remaining salt and pepper with next 5 ingredients in a large bowl. Form mixture into 16 two-inch meatballs.

Heat remaining 2 teaspoons of the oil in a large nonstick skillet over medium heat. Add meatballs and sauté 5 minutes, until browned. Add mushrooms and sauté 3 minutes, until tender and releasing juice; add thyme and stir to coat. Pour in beef broth and simmer 3 minutes, until meatballs are cooked through.

Dissolve cornstarch in sherry and add to skillet; simmer 1 minute, until sauce thickens.

Put smashed sweet potatoes onto individual plates and top with meatballs. Spoon mushroom sauce over top and serve.

Nutrition score per serving (4 meatballs, ¼ cup mushroom sauce, ½ cup sweet potatoes): 411 calories, 24% fat (11 g; 3 g sat.), 44% carbs (45 g), 32% protein (33 g), 66 mg calcium, 4 mg iron, 5 g fiber, 623 mg sodium.

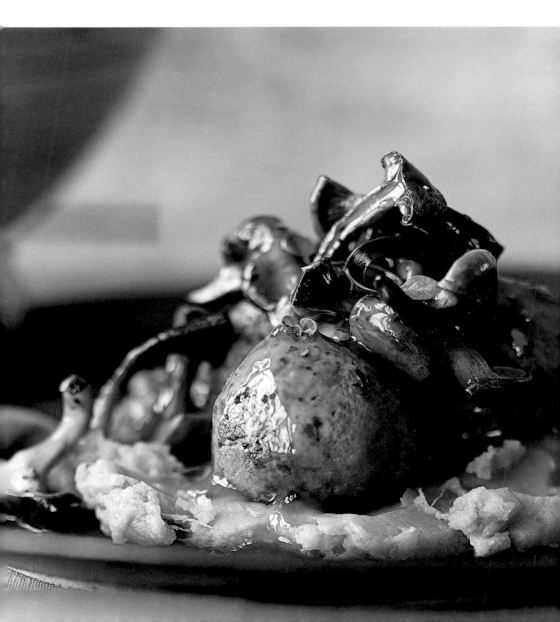

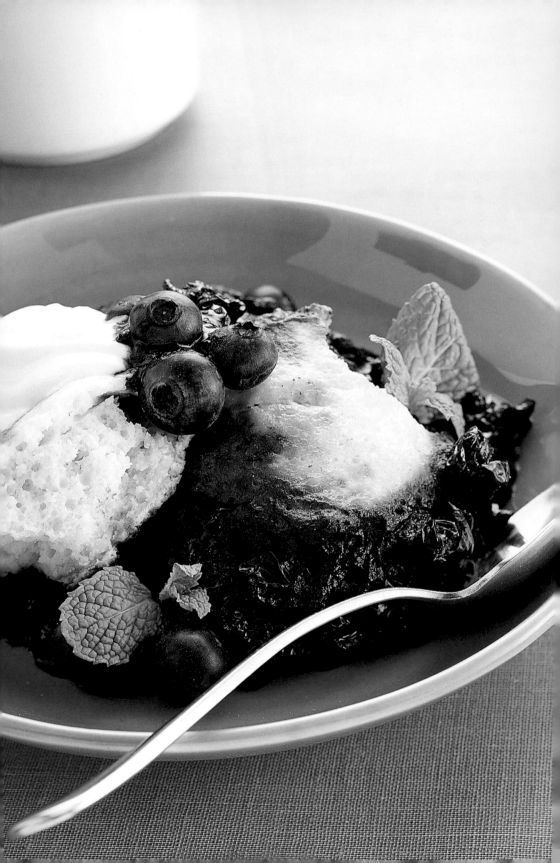

Dumpling-Topped Blueberries

Serves 4
Prep time: 10 minutes
Cook time: 15 minutes

3 cups fresh blueberries
½ cup water
2 tablespoons confectioners' sugar
1 cup all-purpose flour
2 tablespoons granulated sugar
1 teaspoon baking powder
¼ teaspoon salt
¾ cup nonfat milk
½ cup fat-free liquid egg substitute
1 cup nonfat vanilla yogurt

In a large saucepan, combine blueberries, water, and confectioners' sugar. Set pan over high heat and bring to a boil; then reduce heat to medium and simmer 5 minutes.

Meanwhile, in a medium bowl, whisk together flour, granulated sugar, baking powder, and salt. In a small bowl, whisk together milk and egg substitute, and then add to flour mixture; stir until combined.

Using a ½-cup measure, pour 4 heaping half-cups of batter into blueberry mixture to form dumplings (most of the batter will sink to the bottom). Cover pan and simmer 10 minutes without lifting the lid. Check dumplings for doneness (they should be firm and dry to the touch). If not done, replace lid and cook 5 minutes longer. Spoon dumplings and blueberry mixture into shallow bowls and top each serving with ¼ cup yogurt.

Nutrition score per serving (1 dumpling, ¼ cup blueberry mixture, and ¼ cup yogurt): 276 calories, 3% fat (<1 g; 0 g sat.), 80% carbs (55 g), 17% protein (12 g), 231 mg calcium, 2 mg iron, 4 g fiber, 370 mg sodium.

Low-Fat Brownies

Serves: 15
Prep time: 10 minutes
Cook time: 35–40 minutes

Parchment paper
Nonfat cooking spray
¾ cup white sugar
¾ cup dark-brown sugar
½ cup plus 2 tablespoons unsweetened dark-cocoa powder
2 whole eggs
4 egg whites
1¼ cups prunes, pureed in a blender or food processor
    with ½ cup warm water
½ teaspoon salt
½ teaspoon baking soda
½ cup white flour
½ cup whole-wheat flour

Preheat oven to 325° F. Line a 9" x 13" baking pan with parchment paper and coat with cooking spray; set aside. Combine sugars, cocoa powder, eggs, and egg whites in an electric-mixer bowl and beat until light and creamy, about 5 minutes. Slowly spoon in pureed prunes and beat on low until completely mixed in, about 1 minute; add vanilla and salt and mix 30 seconds more. Sift baking soda and flours together and stir lightly into the batter by hand until just absorbed (do not overmix).

Pour into prepared pan and bake 35–40 minutes, until brownies are still soft (but not liquid) in the center. Cool thoroughly and cut into 2" x 2" squares.

Nutrition score per serving (1 brownie): 148 calories, 8% fat (1.41 g; 0.6 g sat.), 82% carbs (33 g), 10% protein (4 g), 15 mg calcium, 1 mg iron, 2 g fiber, 127 mg sodium.

Five- to Ten-Minute
Side Dishes

Mixed-Bean Salad
(Serve alongside grilled chicken or fish)

In a bowl, combine ½ cup each canned red, black, and white beans (rinsed and drained); 1 tablespoon red wine vinegar; 2 teaspoons minced fresh parsley; and 1 teaspoon olive oil. Season with salt and black pepper. Serves 2.

Nutrition score per serving 196 calories, 13% fat (3 g; <1 g sat.), 63% carbs (31 g), 24% protein (12 g), 66 mg calcium, 4 mg iron, 10 g fiber, 5 mg sodium.

Barley Pilaf
(Serve alongside grilled sirloin or roasted chicken)

Bring 1 cup of water to a boil in a medium saucepan. Add ½ cup quick-cooking barley, reduce heat to low, cover, and simmer 8 minutes, until liquid is absorbed and barley is tender. Stir in ½ cup minced carrots, ¼ cup each raisins and minced red onion, and 2 teaspoons each white vinegar and olive oil; season with salt and black pepper, to taste. Serves 2.

Nutrition score per serving: 248 calories, 18% fat (5 g; <1 g sat.), 74% carbs (46 g), 8% protein (5 g), 25 mg calcium, 1 mg iron, 6 g fiber, 29 mg sodium.

Veggie Soup
(Serve with a whole-grain roll
or with a tuna-salad sandwich)

In a large saucepan, combine 1 cup chopped cabbage, 2 chopped carrots, 1 cup thinly sliced mushrooms, ½ cup canned beans (rinsed and drained, any variety), and 4 cups reduced-sodium chicken or vegetable broth. Set pan over high heat and bring to a boil; reduce heat, cover, and simmer 10 minutes, until veggies are tender. Serves 2.

Nutrition score per serving (2 cups): 125 calories, 4% fat (<1 g; 0 g sat.), 65% carbs (20 g), 31% protein (10 g), 50 mg calcium, 2 mg iron, 7 g fiber, 930 mg sodium.

Smoothies for Energy

High-nutrient, creamy shakes are a convenient breakfast or snack that will give you the "get up and go" that you need all day long. Registered dietitian Therese Ann Franzese, M.S., R.D., director of nutrition for the Sports Center at Chelsea Piers in New York City, suggests using only the smoothie ingredients that give you the most nutrition bang for your buck. "Wheat germ is a good additive because it has fiber and protein," she says. "And although it's a fat, flaxseed oil doesn't have any taste and is a great source of valuable omega-3 fatty acids." Other ingredients to keep on hand are unsweetened frozen fruit, blackstrap molasses, low-fat yogurt, low-fat silken tofu, unsweetened-cocoa powder, peanut butter, and blanched whole almonds.

Note: In the recipes that serve two, it's best to make the entire recipe and freeze the rest when you only want one serving. If you reduce the ingredient amounts, you'll lose the smoothie's creamy consistency. When you're ready to have the leftover portion, defrost it for about 10 minutes, then blend for about 40 seconds or until smooth.

Piña Colada Pick-Me-Up

Serve 2
Prep time: 5 minutes

½ cup low-fat silken tofu
¾ cup frozen pineapple chunks
½ cup low-fat coconut- or piña-colada-flavored yogurt
1 tablespoon flaxseed oil
¼ teaspoon coconut extract
⅓ cup water

In a blender, combine tofu and pineapple chunks on "whip" setting for about 20 seconds, until well mixed. Add yogurt, flaxseed oil, coconut extract, and water; continue to whip for 15 seconds.

Nutrition score per serving (7 ounces): 132 calories, 45% fat (7 g; 0.65 g sat.), 49% carbs (16 g), 6% protein (2 g), 292 mg calcium, 0.4 mg iron, 0.6 g fiber, 33 mg sodium.

Avocado Energizer

Serves 2
Prep time: 5 minutes

¼ cup fresh mashed avocado
½ cup low-fat milk
1 teaspoon honey
1 banana, frozen and then broken into 3 pieces
½ cup frozen mango pieces
⅓ cup peach nectar (such as After the Fall or Knudsen)

In a blender, whip together avocado and milk. Add honey, banana, and mango and continue to whip for 10 seconds. Add peach nectar and mix for 5 seconds.

Nutrition score per serving (7 ounces): 207 calories, 27% fat (7 g; 1.6 g sat.), 67% carbs (68 g), 6% protein (4 g), 89 mg calcium, 0.7 mg iron, 3.9 g fiber, 36 mg sodium.

Berry Blast

Serves 2
Prep time: 10 minutes

½ cup frozen sliced or whole strawberries
½ cup low-fat silken tofu
½ cup frozen blueberries
½ cup frozen raspberries
¼ cup low-cal cranberry juice
¼ teaspoon vanilla extract
2 tablespoons wheat germ
1 tablespoon sugar

Allow frozen strawberries to defrost slightly (about 7 minutes on the countertop or 20 seconds in microwave on "defrost").

Meanwhile, in a blender, mix tofu, blueberries, and raspberries on whip setting for 10 seconds. Add strawberries and continue to whip for 5 seconds; put in remaining ingredients and whip for 5 seconds.

Nutrition score per serving (8 ounces): 141 calories, 9% fat (1 g; 0.07 g sat.), 72% carbs (26 g), 19% protein (7 g), 45 mg calcium, 1.7 mg iron, 6 g fiber, 59 mg sodium.

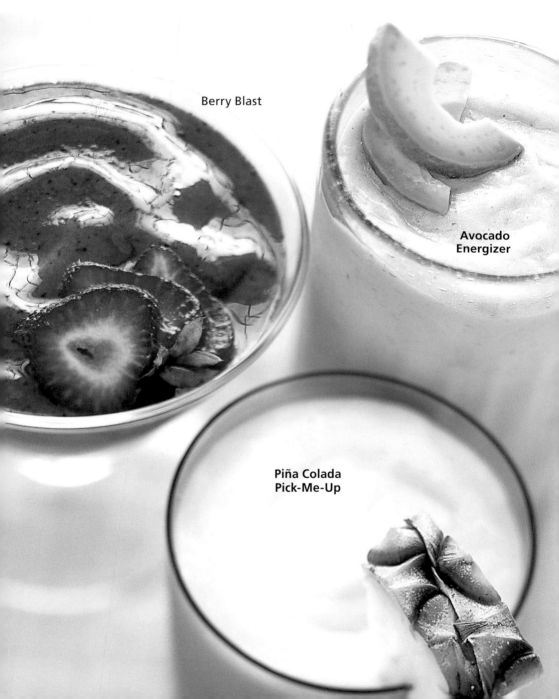

Berry Blast

Avocado
Energizer

Piña Colada
Pick-Me-Up

Chocolate Charge

Serves 1
Prep time: 5 minutes

½ cup crushed ice (about 8 cubes)
1 tablespoon unsweetened-cocoa powder
¼ teaspoon vanilla extract
1 tablespoon blackstrap molasses
¼ cup low-fat milk
1 cup low-fat vanilla frozen yogurt
1 teaspoon crushed almonds

Combine ice, cocoa powder, vanilla, molasses, and milk; blend on high for about 10 seconds or until smooth. Add frozen yogurt and blend for 5 more seconds. You might top with crushed almonds.

Nutrition score per serving (7 ounces): 189 calories, 21% fat (4.6 g; 2 g sat.), 67% carbs (33 g), 12% protein (6 g), 290 mg calcium, 3 mg iron, 1 g fiber, 122 mg sodium.

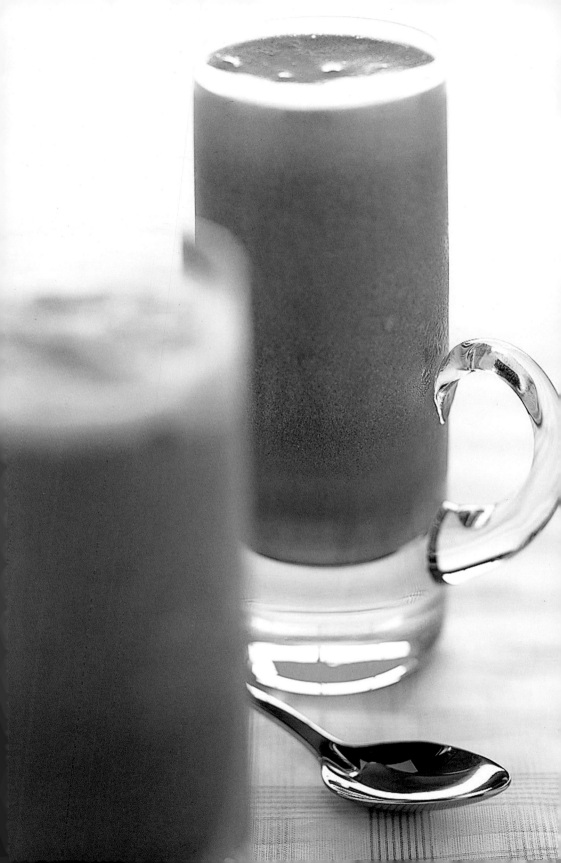

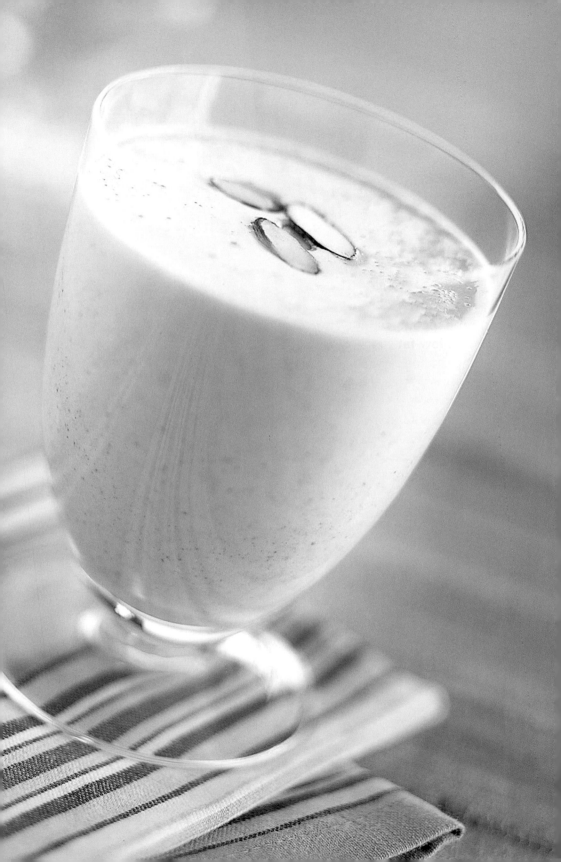

Peanut Butter Power-Up

Serves 1
Prep time: 5 minutes

1 tablespoon peanut butter
½ cup low-fat vanilla frozen yogurt
1 tablespoon slivered or sliced blanched almonds
2 teaspoons flaxseed oil
¼ teaspoon almond extract
⅓ cup low-fat milk

In a blender, mix peanut butter and frozen yogurt on whip for about 5 seconds. Add almonds, flaxseed oil, and almond extract and whip for 5 seconds; pour in milk and whip for 5 seconds.

Nutrition score per serving (7 ounces): 369 calories, 57% fat (26 g; 5 g sat.), 31% carbs (32 g), 12% protein (12 g), 272 mg calcium, 0.7 mg iron, 1.9 g fiber, 213 mg sodium.

Ultimate Word

One of the most important things you can do to achieve your Ultimate Body is to eat your veggies. Sometimes you can find crafty ways to sneak them into your diet. Here are some painless techniques for helping you make your daily quota:

- Slip ¼ cup of spinach, arugula, or watercress leaves into a turkey sandwich.

- Use finely chopped spinach anywhere you'd find herbs, such as in pasta or potato salads.

- Add shredded raw zucchini or carrots to cookie, muffin, or quick-bread batter.

- Blend a cup of raw grated carrots or squash into your favorite meat-loaf recipe.

- Substitute steamed turnips, rutabagas, or celery root for half of your mashed potatoes.

- Puree steamed cauliflower with a few Tablespoons of broth, and use to thicken sauces.

- Replace lasagna noodles with eggplant slices, which have a similar texture.

We hope these recipes and tips have left you feeling energized and invigorated. With the right fuel and our powerhouse exercise programs, you're well on the way to your Ultimate Body . . . enjoy the journey!

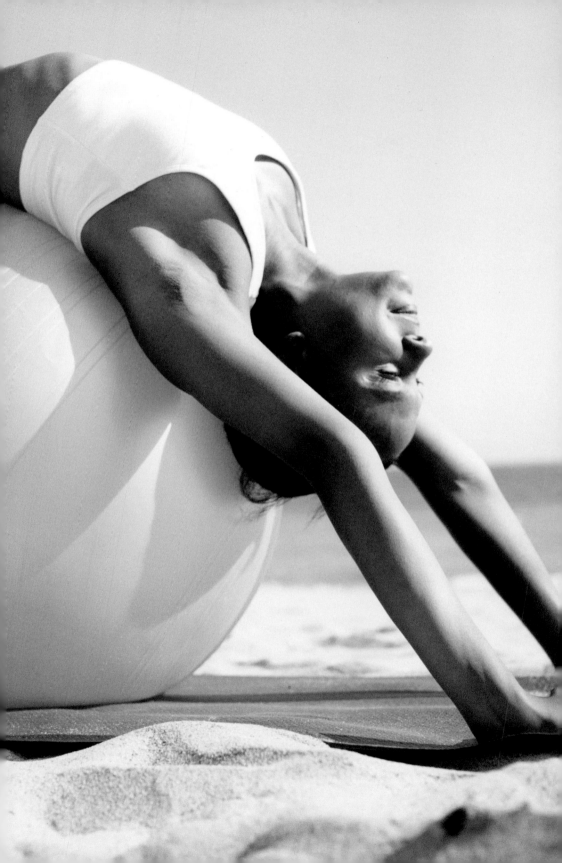

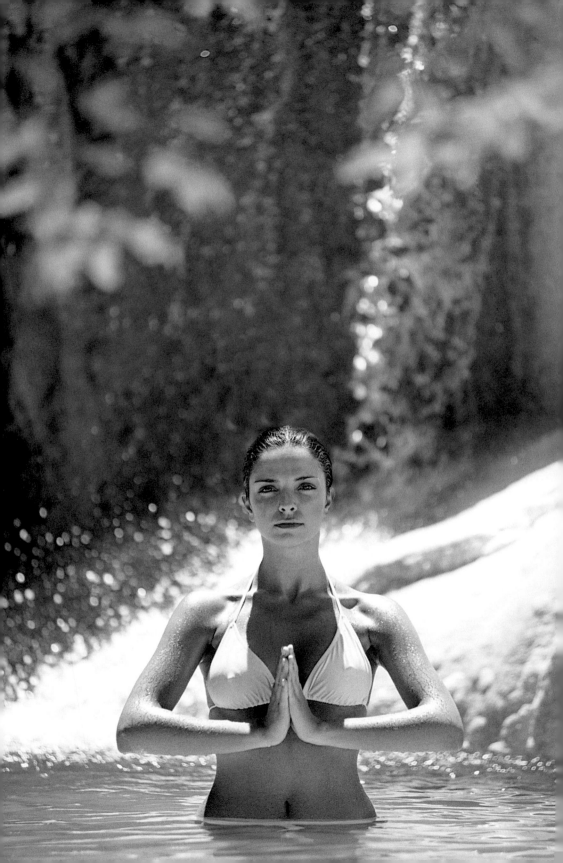

Contributors

We'd like to gratefully acknowledge and thank all of the writers whose articles, which first appeared in *Shape* magazine, are now used in this book:

Karen Asp, "Too Hot to Trot?" August 2003

Sarah Bowen Shea, "Maximum Results, Minimum Time," June 2004

Beverly Burmeier, "Eat Like a Kid Again," May 2004

Susan Cantwell, "Use Guilt to Catapult You Forward," December 2000

Connie Chow, "Don't Drown the Veggies," March 2004

Alona Friedman, "Breaking Up (with Your Trainer) Is Hard to Do," September 2004

Ramin Ganeshram, "Smoothies for Energy," May 2003; "Heart-y Lowfat Valentine Brownies," February 2004.

Brenda Goodman, "5 Crucial Stats for Weight Loss," March 2005

Angela Hynes, "Are You Really Ready?" March 2004

Lisa Jhung, "Workout Equipment Q & A," April 2003

Patricia King, "When You're the New Kid in Gym Class," September 2004

Valerie Latona, "Life in Balance," December 2002

Lorie A. Parch, "Gym-Goer, Beware," March 2005

Carol Potera, "Workout Motivation: Will You Be Back?" July 2004; "The Sedentary American," October 2004

Suzanne Schlosberg, "No Excuses Workout," November 2000; "Short Circuit," August 2003; "Fitness Q & A," September 2004

Jenna Schnuer, "The Post-Binge Diet," February 2004

Linda Shelton, "Life in Balance," December 2002; "Blast Your Ab Flab," December 2003; "Sculpted Lean and Serene," September 2004

Alexa Joy Sherman, "Best Butt," September 2002; "The Secrets to Strength-Training Success," June 2003; "5-Minute Fitness," November 2003; "Bikini Ready (in 8 Weeks)," May 2004; "Total Body Power Yoga," November 2004

Emily Shroeder, "Walk or Run Your Butt Off!" March 2003

Jacqueline Stenson, "Beat the Bonk!" March 2004

Tracy Teare, "Six Tips to Take the Weight Off," March 2003; "Age Defying Workout," October, 2004

Robin Vitetta Miller, M.S., "Shop Till You Drop (Pounds)," May 2002; "Recipe of the Month—Blueberry Slump," June 2003; "Eat Your Good Carbs," October 2003; "Make Over Your Kitchen to Lose Weight," January 2004; "Filling Snacks to Pack," September 2004

Amanda Vogel, "What the Heck Is 'Neutral' Posture?" July 2004

Stacy Whitman, "30-Minute Total-Body Workout," December 2001; "Maximum Results at Home . . . or at the Gym," September 2002; "One-Minute Workouts," November 2002; "Surprising Secrets to Cardio Success," February 2003; "Overhaul Your Ball Workout," May 2003; "Get a Better Butt," November 2003; "The Ultimate At-Home Exercise Guide," December 2004

Photo Credits

Photography: Nick Horne • *Hair:* Sonia Lee/Artists Management Inc. • *Makeup:* Mauricio Lemus for Beauty & Photo • *Styling:* Dinah Erasmus • *On-set styling:* Zoe Joeright/Artists by Timothy Priano • *Producer:* Nancy Leopardi for **LAphotoProducer.com**

Front Cover: *Woman boxing:* Ron Cadiz, August 2004; *woman reaching up:* Willie Maldonado, December 2003; *woman on ball with weights:* Larry Bartholomew, May 2003; *woman with hands on hips:* Dorian Castor, January 2004

James Allen, "30-Minute Total Body Workout," December 2001

Mario de Lopez, "30-Day Total Body Makeover," April 2002

David Price, "Shop Till You Drop," May 2002

Beatriz da Costa, "3 Easy Ways to Cook Low-Fat," June 2002

Willie Maldonado, "Workouts for Best Butt," September 2002

James Allen, "Get Maximum Results at Home or the Gym," September 2002

Adam Brown, "The Best Workout for Weight Loss," October 2002

Willie Maldonado, "One-Minute Workouts," November 2002

Shannon Greer, "Surprising Secrets to Cardio Success," February 2003

Lisa Loftus, "Walk or Run your Butt Off," March 2003

Pornchai Mittongtare, "Smoothies for Energy," May 2003

Larry Bartholomew, "Overhaul Your Ball Workout," May 2003

Shannon Greer, "Secrets to Strength Training Success," June 2003

David Prince, "Recipe of the Month: Blueberry Slump," June 2003

Marc Addleman, "Short Circuit," August 2003

Luca Trocato, "Eat Your Good Carbs," October 2003

James Allen, "5-Minute Fitness," November 2003

Willie Maldonado, "Blast Your Ab Flab," December 2003

Pascal Demeester, "Your Best Lower Body in Only 30 Days," January 2004

Dorian Caster, "What's Your Goal," January 2004

Lisa Hubbard, "Make Over Your Kitchen," January 2004

Roni Ramos, Still-Life Photography, "Make Over Your Kitchen," January 2004

Willie Maldonado, "The Body-Sculpting, Fat-Blasting, No-Burnout Workout," February 2004

Dominick Guilemot, "Bikini Ready in 8 Weeks," May 2004

Willie Maldonado, "Maximum Result, Minimum Time," June 2004

Robert Deutschman, "Sculpted, Lean and Serene," September 2004

Nick Horne, "Your At-Home Yoga Guide," September 2004

James Allen, "Total Body Power Yoga," November 2004

Larry Bartholomew, "At Home Poster with accompanying gym program-same body parts gym moves," December 2004

Ron Cadiz, " Core Training for Your Best Body," August 2004

Illustrations: Karen Kuchar • *Photo research:* Christina Cummins

About the Authors

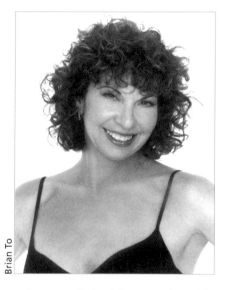

Brian To

Linda Shelton has served as the fitness director for *Shape* magazine for 21 years, and she also oversees the fitness sections for *Fit Pregnancy* and *Natural Health* magazines. She's an internationally recognized fitness trainer, lecturer, and health writer with 35 years of teaching experience in the exercise field. A frequent guest on television and radio talk shows, Linda has appeared on programs including *Good Morning America,* E! Entertainment Television, and *Inside Edition.* She's the author of *The Method Jump Start Journal: 8 Weeks to Wellness,* and has written two books with premier personal trainer Keli Roberts: *Fitness Hollywood* and *Stronger Legs and Lower Body.*

She has worked as a producer, director, fitness consultant/technical advisor, scriptwriter, and/or choreographer for more than 250 fitness videos, including *Shape*'s DVD workout series, *Platinum Series: Buns of Steel 2000, Crunch Fitness* series, and the *Dummies* video line. Linda enjoys hiking with her two golden retrievers, gardening, dancing, and weight training; and she still teaches yoga, strength, and Pilates classes regularly.

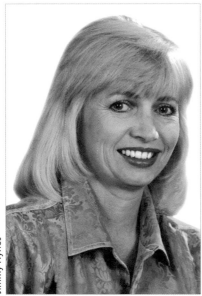

Jimmy Hynes

Angela Hynes is a freelance writer and editor specializing in health and fitness. She's the co-author of *Shape Your Life* (with Barbara Harris), a regular contributor to *Shape*, and a contributing editor to *Natural Health* magazine; her work has also appeared in numerous other national and international publications. A resident of Los Angeles, she exercises every day and enjoys hiking in the local hills. She's also an adventure-travel enthusiast.

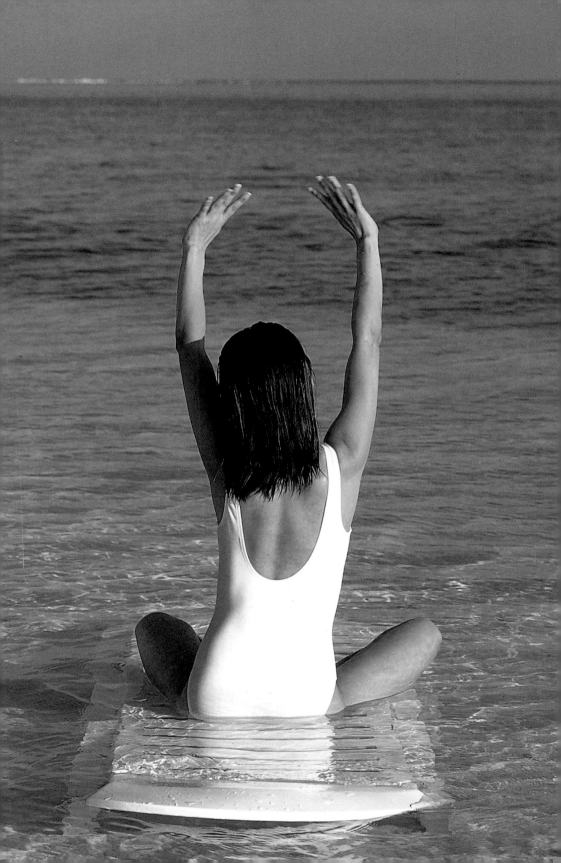

We hope you enjoyed this Hay House book.
If you'd like to receive a free catalog featuring additional
Hay House books and products, or if you'd like information
about the Hay Foundation, please contact:

Hay House, Inc.
P.O. Box 5100
Carlsbad, CA 92018-5100

(760) 431-7695 or **(800) 654-5126**
(760) 431-6948 (fax) or **(800) 650-5115 (fax)**
www.hayhouse.com

Published and distributed in Australia by:
Hay House Australia Pty. Ltd. • 18/36 Ralph St. • Alexandria NSW
2015 • *Phone:* 612-9669-4299 • *Fax:* 612-9669-4144
www.hayhouse.com.au

Published and distributed in the United Kingdom by:
Hay House UK, Ltd. • Unit 62, Canalot Studios
222 Kensal Rd., London W10 5BN • *Phone:* 44-20-8962-1230
Fax: 44-20-8962-1239 • www.hayhouse.co.uk

Published and distributed in the Republic of South Africa by:
Hay House SA (Pty), Ltd., P.O. Box 990, Witkoppen 2068
Phone/Fax: 27-11-706-6612 • orders@psdprom.co.za

Distributed in Canada by:
Raincoast • 9050 Shaughnessy St., Vancouver, B.C. V6P 6E5
Phone: (604) 323-7100 • *Fax:* (604) 323-2600

Tune in to **www.hayhouseradio.com**™ for the best in
inspirational talk radio featuring top Hay House authors!
And, sign up via the Hay House USA Website to receive the
Hay House online newsletter and stay informed about what's
going on with your favorite authors. You'll receive bimonthly
announcements about: Discounts and Offers, Special Events,
Product Highlights, Free Excerpts, Giveaways, and more!
www.hayhouse.com

SUBSCRIBE to **SHAPE** today a
take your fitness even further!

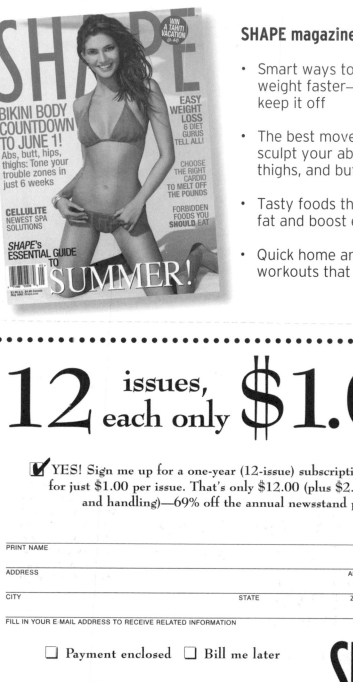

SHAPE magazine shows you:

- Smart ways to lose weight faster—and keep it off

- The best moves to sculpt your abs, thighs, and butt

- Tasty foods that blast fat and boost energy

- Quick home and gym workouts that get results

ou don't want to miss what's new in every issue of **SHAPE!**

- Target training exercise cards

- Pull-out posters

- Success stories

And more!

Start getting SHAPE in your mailbox. Fill out and mail the attached card now—or subscribe at **www.shapeinfo.com**